AF572298

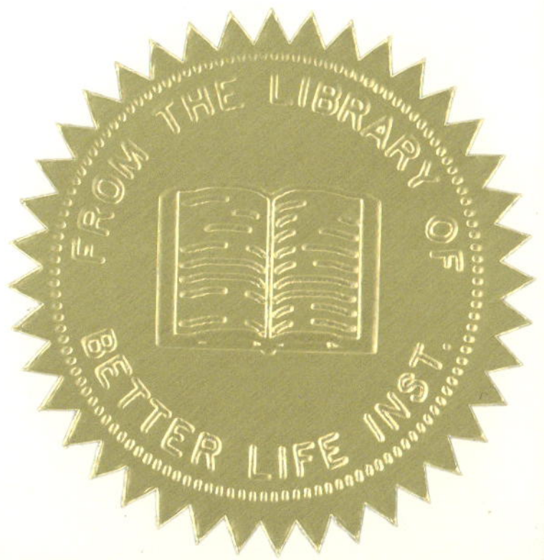
FROM THE LIBRARY OF
BETTER LIFE INST.

Preventive Cardiology

Preventive Cardiology

Proceedings of an International Symposium held
at Billingehus, Skövde, Sweden
August 21st, 1971
under the Sponsorship of the Planning Group
for Preventive Cardiology of the Swedish Medical
Research Council

Edited by

GÖSTA TIBBLIN, ANCEL KEYS and LARS WERKÖ

Almqvist & Wiksell
Stockholm

A Halsted Press Book
John Wiley & Sons
New York – London – Sydney – Toronto

Almqvist & Wiksell ISBN 91-20-03112-2

Wiley ISBN 0-470-86760-4
Library of Congress Catalog Card Number 72–4152

Printed in Sweden by
Almqvist & Wiksell Informationsindustri AB, Uppsala 1972

Foreword

On the official WHO-list of age-specific death rates for cardiovascular diseases Sweden is rather down the scale in Europe. When we consider the major causes of death however cardiovascular diseases, dominate the picture. Therefore it is natural to take measures in an effort to control these very common diseases. An important step was then the establishment of a Planning Group in Preventive Cardiology under the auspices of the Swedish Medical Research Council. The aim was to start heart control programs in different areas of Sweden.

In association with the Council on Epidemiology and Prevention of the International Society of Cardiology the Planning Group organized this symposium on Preventive Cardiology.

The proceedings of the symposium are published with the feeling that their usefulness will not be limited to those interested in one particular report. It is hoped that the volume also will attract those readers who are interested in the general problem of benefits and drawbacks of prevention of heart diseases.

As the organizers of the symposium it is our privilege to thank all those having made possible this conference and the publication of the proceedings. Our sincere thanks are directed towards the contributors to this volume and to our collaborators at the Section of Preventive Cardiology, Department of Internal Medicine, Sahlgren's hospital, Göteborg, who all supported the enterprises in connection with this meeting. (They are Drs. Lars Wilhelmsson, Dag Elmfeldt, Anders Vedin and Claes Wilhelmsson.) The Swedish Medical Research Council and "National Association against Heart and Lung Disease" have generously sponsered the conference. Mrs Inga-Lisa Ljungberg has been our most efficient secretary at this meeting.

G. T. L. W.

Contents

Foreword 5
List of participants 9
L. Werkö
Welcoming address 11
J. Stamler
The challenges and possibilities for prevention in mass community efforts to control the major coronary risk factors 13

Part I
Risk factors for ischemic heart disease
Chairman: *L. Werkö*
A. Keys
Predicting coronary heart disease 21
G. Tibblin
Risk factors for developing myocardial infarction and other diseases. The "Men born in 1913" study 33
J. Stamler
The National Cooperative Pooling Project in the United States . 43
H. Blackburn, P. Canner, W. Krol, S. Tominaga and J. Stamler
The natural history of myocardial infarction in the Coronary Drug Project. Prognostic indicators following infarction 54
Discussion:
Risk factors—cause or effect? 65

Part II
Changing risk factors
Chairman: *G. Biörck*
P. Leren
Lipid reduction by diet 75
P. From Hansen
Lipid reduction by drugs 79
B. Hood
Antihypertensive treatment and myocardial infarction 83
G. Rose
Anti-smoking programmes 92

L. Wilhelmsen
A smoking cessation program in a field trial 97
M. J. Karvonen
Physical inactivity 103
Discussion
Preventive approach to cardiovascular diseases–benefits and drawbacks 108

Part III
Heart control programme
Chairman: *J. Morris*
Z. Pisa
The WHO heart control programme in Europe 117
V. Kallio
The heart control programme in Finland 124
G. Tibblin
The heart control programme in Sweden 127
D. Elmfeldt and L. Wilhelmsen
A study of representative post myocardial infarction patients aged 27–55 129
C. Bengtsson
Myocardial infarction in young women 140
P. Harmsen, G. Berglund, O. Larsson, S. Sörenson and G. Tibblin
The Stroke Register in Göteborg 148
H. Sanne, D. Elmfeldt and L. Wilhelmsen
Preventive effect of physical training after a myocardial infarction 154
J. A. Vedin and C. E. Wilhelmsson
Evaluation of a myocardial infarction out-patient clinic–A Secondary Preventive Trial 161
G. Dahlén, C. Ericson, C. Furberg, L. Lundkvist and K. Svärdsudd
Lipoprotein pattern in IHD 166
S. O. Isacsson
Calf blood flow and smoking 171
General discussion 180

List of participants

Bengtsson, Calle, Department of Medicine II, Sahlgren's hospital, Göteborg, Sweden

Biörck, Gunnar, Department of Medicine, Serafimerlasarettet, Stockholm, Sweden

Bjurö, Thorvald, Department of Rehabilitation, Sahlgren's hospital, Göteborg, Sweden

Blackburn, Henry, Laboratory of Physiological Hygiene University of Minnesota Minneapolis, Minnesota, USA

Carlsson, Lars A., Department for Geriatrics. Uppsala University, Uppsala, Sweden

Elmfeldt, Dag, Department of Medicine II, Sahlgren's hospital, Göteborg, Sweden

Furberg, Curt, Laboratory of Clinical Physiology, Boden county hospital, Boden, Sweden

Hansen, Per From, Københavns Amtssygehus, Glostrup, Danmark

Harmsen, Per, Department of Neurology, Sahlgren's hospital, Göteborg, Sweden

Hedstrand, Hans, Department of Medicine, Akademiska sjukhuset, Uppsala, Sweden

Hofvendahl, Stefan, Department of Medicine, Serafimerlasarettet, Stockholm, Sweden

Hood, Bertil, Department of Medicine, Lund University, Lund, Sweden

Isacsson, Sven-Olof, Department of Social Medicine, Malmö City Hospital, Malmö, Sweden

Jakobsson, Sören, Department of Medicine, Gävle County hospital, Gävle, Sweden

Johansson, Bengt V., Department of Medicine, Malmö City hospital, Malmö, Sweden

Kallio, Veikko, Department of Medicine, County hospital Åbo, Åbo, Finland

Karvonen, Martti J., Institute of Occupational Health, Haartimaninkatu 1, Helsinki 25, Finland

Keys, Ancel, Laboratory of Physiological Hygiene, University of Minnesota, Minneapolis, Minnesota, USA

Korsgren, Magnus, Department of Medicine, Falun County hospital, Falun, Sweden

Leren, Paul, Ullevål Sykehus, Oslo, Norge

Morris, Jerry, London School of Hygiene and Tropical Medicine, London, Great Britain

Mulcahy, R., Coronary Heart Disease Research Unit, St. Vincent's hospital, Dublin Ireland

Pisa, Z., Regional Officer for Chronic Diseases, WHO, Dk-2100 Copenhagen, Danmark

Remington, Richard, School of Public Health at Houston, The University of Texas, Houston, Texas, USA

Rose, Geoffrey, London School of Hygiene and Tropical Medicine, London, Great Britain

Sanne, Harald, Department of Rehabilitation, Sahlgren's hospital, Göteborg, Sweden

Stamler, Jeremiah, Council on Epidemiology and Prevention, International Society of Cardiology, Chicago Civic Center, Chicago, Illinois, USA

Stamler, Rose, Chicago Civic Center, Chicago, Illinois, USA

Taylor, Henry, Laboratory of Physiological Hygiene, University of Minnesota, Minneapolis, Minnesota, USA

Tibblin, Gösta, Department of Medicine I, Sahlgren's hospital, Göteborg, Sweden

Vedin, Anders, Department of Medicine I, Sahlgren's hospital, Göteborg, Sweden

Werkö, Lars, Department of Medicine I, Sahlgren's hospital, Göteborg, Sweden

Wilhelmsen, Lars, Department of Medicine I, Sahlgren's hospital, Göteborg, Sweden

Welcoming address

by Lars Werkö

The Council of Epidemiology of the International Society for Cardiology has made a concentrated effort to increase the knowledge regarding cardiovascular epidemiology all around the world. One very important part of this effort has been the yearly courses of epidemiology that has seen held in August or September in some parts of Europe. This year Sweden was selected as host for this course and we deemed it natural to grasp the opportunity and arrange a conference on preventive cardiology where we could update the situation having so many eminent scientists from all over the world with us.

In this setting I do not need to dwell on the importance of the problem facing us. Most of you have been so deeply involved during so many years that you may be somewhat astonished to hear that the Swedish authorities have not quite understood the magnitude of the impact of the cardiovascular diseases on the society, both outside the hospitals and for the clinical medicine proper, until lately.

However, two years ago the Swedish Medical Research Council created a committee on preventive cardiology with the aim of increasing and coordinating the efforts of combating cardiovascular diseases in the society, especially ischemic heart disease. This conference is sponsored by this committee as well as by the Swedish Association against Heart and Lung disease. The whole project had not started had it not been for the efforts of WHO, that especially in Europe has had a comprehensive programme running for the last couple of years. Much of the presentations today will center around that programme.

The real missionaries for the cause of international cooperation within this field are also with us during this time and it gives me great pleasure to welcome Ancel Keys and Jerry Stamler among us. Without their dedicated work neither international cardiovascular epidemiology nor the ISC Council had occupied the firm position it now has. The present chairman of the international council. Jerry Morris, is representing the council but to a much larger extent himself and the British Medical Research Council. Similarly we are happy to have amongst us Zbynek Pisa, who has been of such importance for the European WHO Control Programme.

I have mentioned a few people in this introduction. This does not mean that you are not all equally welcome. We are very happy that you all have been able to come and hope that you will take part in to-days deliberations with the same intensity that I am quite sure that for example Jerry Stamler will do. So let's start with our formal programme.

You may think that we have been a little provocative using as title for the coming panel discussion "risk factors, cause or effect?" This was done in order to have a good starting point for a real debate not only of the import of serum cholesterol and high blood pressure, cigarette smoking and physical inactivity in predicting the future event of myocardial infarction but also of factors like psychosocial instability, status incongruity, personality types and other less studied variables.

There are several problems that still need solution—some of them even a well formulated hypothesis. Let me list a few that we may address us to.

Is the serum cholesterol the best predictive factor for IHD?

And is the reduction of serum cholesterol the most important presentive measures that we should aim at?

What about other lipids?

What is the situation of the "water story"?

How does smoking cigarettes enter the predictive picture in different part of the world?

What is the significance of psychosocial circumstances? And do they act by themselves—through neural or humoral pathways—or through more ordinary metabolic mechanisms?

Is the final catastrophe of a myocardial infaction due to *one* or to a set of factors acting throughout a life time? Or is there one set of events leeding to vascular disease and another acting on top of the former to release the killing blow to the myocardium?

Has the day come for a general preventive effort? If so, how should this be organized?

You can comprehend that we have quite a lot to discuss so let's start with some facts collected in several international or national studies.

The challenges and possibilities for prevention in mass community efforts to control the major coronary risk factors

By Jeremiah Stamler

The challenges and possibilities inherent in mass screening to detect coronary-prone persons – the implications for the effort to curb the coronary epidemic – can be fully comprehended and appreciated only when considered in the light of specific and concrete facts. In my later presentation, I will cite the data available from the U.S. National Cooperative Pooling Project on the impact of the three major coronary risk factors, singly and in combination (1, 2, 2a–l). It is relevant to our present theme to examine the data once again, this time in terms of the potential for prevention. While this is U.S. experience, it clearly is meaningful for other countries, at least the industrialized ones.

Let us examine the risk factors one by one, beginning with hypertension. At the present in the USA of all the hypertensives – totalling 20 to 25 million persons – almost half are undetected. Of the half who realize they are hypertensive, about half are receiving no treatment. Of the remaining quarter, about half are being treated inadequately, so that they remain hypertensive (3–7). Given this situation with regard to undetected, untreated, and inadequately treated high blood pressure, the rough estimate is that only about one-eighth – 1/2 x 1/2 x 1/2 – of the U.S. hypertensives are being given sufficient treatment to lower their blood pressure appeciably, i. e., to diastolic level less than 95 mm. Hg.

Let us assume that the level of effective treatment can be increased to embrace 50 per cent of the hypertensives, and let us explore the possible consequences, in terms of mortality from coronary heart disease and all causes for men age 30–59 of the type studied in the Pooling Project. The age-adjusted ten-year CHD death rate for these men with diastolic pressure $\geqslant$ 95 mm. Hg at entry was 54 per 1 000; the all causes mortality rate, 109. Let us assume that the CHD mortality rate of the well-treated hypertensives can be lowered from 54 to 30 per 1 000, a reduction of 44,4 per cent. This rate of 30 per 1 000 is still above that of the normotensive subgroups (26 and 20 per 1 000). From the limited experience of the U.S. Veterans Administration Cooperative Study on Antihypertensive Agents, this is a reasonable estimate of effectiveness of therapy (1, 8). It is reasonable to make a further assumption as to effectiveness of antihypertensive treatment against cardiovascular mortality overall–e. g., against stroke, in addition to CHD–so that all causes mortality for the well-treated hypertensives is lowered to 70 per 1 000. This would mean a lowering of the all causes death rate of 35.6 per cent for the hypertensives, once again, a reasonable assumption (1, 8). For the total population of men age 30–59, the net result of effectively treating half the hypertensives (i. e., just under 10 per cent of the total population) would be a reduction in overall CHD mortality rate of 6.3 per cent, from 32 per 1 000 to 30 per 1 000, and a reduction of all causes mortality rate of 5.6 per cent, from 72 to 68 per 1 000. Lest these decreases seem insignificant, I hasten to add that no improvement in life expectancy for middle-aged white American males has occurred in the 20th centuty (9). A 5.6 per cent reduction in all causes mortality for the 35 million U.S. men age 30–59 would mean saving of about 14 000 lives per year!

A similar set of calculations can readily be made as to the estimated gains from a successful effort to reduce the proportion of men in the population who are cigarette smokers. Let us estimate the consequences of converting 30 per cent of current cigarette smokers, again men age 30–59, to ex-smokers, with a ten-year CHD mortality rate reduced to 24 per 1 000, and an all causes death rate to 46 per 1 000, rates for men smoking pipe and/or cigars only. For these reformed cigarette smokers, this would represent a decrease in CHD mortality rate of 40.0 per cent, and in all causes mortality rate of 50.0 per cent. For the total population, this would be a decrease in CHD mortality rate of 12.5 per cent, and in all causes mortality rate of 11.3 per cent. This would mean an annual saving of about 30 000 lives among the 30 million U.S. men age 30–59. No wonder that public health experts have characterized a successful mass campaign against cigarette smoking as the single most important thing that could be done to improve life expectancy in the industrialized countries.

Let us repeat the calculations, now estimating the fruits of a successful effort to identify 50 per cent of U.S. hypercholesterolemic men ($\geqslant$ 250 mg./dl.) and lower their serum cholesterol by 10 per cent by safe feasible nutritional procedures (1, 10–12). Previous calculations permit the estimate of a 24.4 per cent lowering of CHD incidence from a 10 per cent reduction in serum cholesterol (1, 14). Let us assume a similar effect on CHD mortality rate. The impact on all causes mortality rate for the 50 per cent of hypercholesterolemic men so influenced nutritionally is projected to be 6.9 per cent, assuming no impact on any other type of atherosclerotic mortality (e. g., stroke) other than CHD (1, 2, 2a–l). For the total population, the net effect on CHD mortality rate would be a reduction of 6.1 per cent, and on mortality from all causes, 2.9 per cent, with a saving of over 7 000 lives per year.

The inference from the prospective epidemiologic studies is that an across-the-board improvement could be attained by fat modification of the diet to lower serum cholesterol of the whole population (1, 2, 2a–l). The National Diet-Heart Study unequivocally demonstrated that such a reduction in serum cholesterol is feasible (11). It is therefore worthwhile to estimate what the effects on mortality rates would be if various proportions of the general population of adult males changed diet habits enough to lower serum cholesterol 10 per cent. Again, let us take the estimate that a 24.4 per cent reduction in CHD mortality would result, with no effect on mortality from severe atherosclerosis of other arterial beds. From the data, it can readily be calculated that if 25 per cent of U.S. white males age 30–59 were to make these changes, the net effect on CHD mortality rate for the population would be a 6.1 per cent reduction, and on all causes mortality rate, a 2.9 per cent reduction. If 50 per cent of U.S. white males age 30–59 were to make these changes in diet habit and serum cholesterol, the net effect on CHD mortality rate for the population would be a 12.2 per cent reduction, and on all causes mortality rate, a 5.7 per cent reduction, with a saving of over 14 000 lives per year.

Finally, let us assess the preventive potential of combined intervention against the three major risk factors (hypertension, cigarette smoking, hypercholesterolemia) in highly coronary-prone men with any two or all three of these dangerous traits. Obviously such an approach has a great deal to recommend it; it makes great public health sense, theoretically and practically (1, 10, 12). Again, let us use the Pooling Project experience as our guide. Note the typical American situation, product of our way of life; only 1 249 of the 7 342 white males age 30–59 at entry –i. e., only 17 per cent–were classified not high for all three factors. All the rest had one or more risk factors; 45 per cent with one, 30 per cent with two, 8 per cent with all three. These latter two subgroups, with any two or all three risk factors (38 % of the total group), accounted for 57 per cent of coronary deaths, 55 per cent of all deaths.

By multifactor intervention, it is reasonable to anticipate a substantial reduction in mortality rates for these very high risk men. The estimates are based on the assumption that both CHD and all causes mortality rates can be reduced by over 50 per cent, to levels slightly below those for men with one risk factor only, but still substantially higher than those for men with none of the three traits. If these changes were successfully accomplished for half these very high risk men, i. e., for about 20 per cent of the population, this would yield an 18.7 per cent net reduction in CHD mortality and a 17.8 per cent reduction in all causes mortality for the total population, with a saving of almost 45 000 lives per year.

These would indeed be substantial achievements, a major turn in life expectancy for U.S. adult males. These then are the stakes–the challenges and possibilities for primary prevention and public health advance–in the projected mass community efforts to control the major coronary risk factors.

References

1. Inter-Society Comission for Heart Disease Resources. Atherosclerosis Study Group and Epidemiology Study Group. Primary Prevention of the Atherosclerotic Diseases. *Circulation, 42,* A55, 1970.
2. Data from the Pooling Project, Council on Epidemiology, American Heart Association–a national cooperative project for pooling data from the Albany civil servant, Chicago Peoples Gas Company, Chicago Western Electric Company, Framingham community, Los Angeles civil servant, Minneapolis-St. Paul business men, and other prospective epidemiologic studies of adult cardiovascular disease in the United States. The following are representative references on the individual studies and on the results of the Pooling Project to date:

2a. Doyle, J. T., Risk Factors in Coronary Heart Disease. *New York State J. Med., 63,* 1317, 1963.

2b. Stamler, J., Cardiovascular Diseases in the United States. *Amer. J. Cardiol., 10,* 319, 1962.

2c. Paul, O., Lepper, M. H., Phelan, W. H., Dupertuis, G. W., MacMillan, A., McKean, H. and Park, H., A Longitudinal Study of Coronary Heart Disease. *Circulation, 28,* 20, 1963.

2d. Dawber, T. R., Kannel, W. B. and McNamara, P. M., The Prediction of Coronary Heart Disease. *Trans. Assoc. Life Insur. Med. Dir. Amer., 47,* 70, 1964.

2e. Chapman, J. M. and Massey, F. J., The Interrelationship of Serum Cholesterol, Hypertension, Body Weight, and Risk of Coronary Disease. Results of the First Ten Years Follow-up in the Los Angeles Heart Study. *J. Chron. Dis., 17,* 933, 1964.

2f. Keys, A., Taylor, H. L., Blackburn, H., Brozek, J., Anderson, J. T. and Simonson, E., Coronary Heart Disease among Minnesota Business and Professional Men Followed Fifteen Years. *Circulation, 28,* 381, 1963.

2g. Moore, F. E., *Some Preliminary Findings from the Pooling Project of the Council on Epidemiology, American Heart Association.* Paper Presented at the Conference on Cardiovascular Disease Epidemiology, Council on Epidemiology, American Heart Association, March 3–4, 1969, New Orleans, La.

2h. Doyle, J. T. and Kinch, S. H., *Coronary Heart Disease in the United States: Some Preliminary Findings from the Pooling Project of the Council on Epidemiology of the American Heart Association.* Presented at the 42nd Scientific Sessions, American Heart Association, Nov. 14, 1969.

2i. Epstein, F. H. and Moore, F. E., Progress Report to the National Heart Institute on the National Cooperative Pooling Project, 1968.

2j. Paul O., The Risk of Mild Hypertension: A Ten Year Report. *Brit. Heart J., 33,* (Suppl.), 116, 1971.

2k. Doyle, J. T. and Kannel, W. B., *Coronary Risk Factors: 10 Year Findings in 7 446 Americans. Pooling Project, Council on Epidemiology, American Heart Association.* Paper Presented at the VI World Congress of Cardiology, London, England, September, 1970.

2l. Berkson, D. M., Stamler, J., Lindberg, H. A., Miller, W. A., Stevens, E. L., Soyugenc, R., Tokich, T. J. and Stamler, R., Heart Rate: An Important Risk Factor for Coronary Mortality–Ten Year Experience of the Peoples Gas Co. Epidemiologic Study (1958–68). Jones, R. J., Ed., *Atherosclerosis,* Second International Symposium, Springer-Verlag, New York, N. Y., 382, 1970.

3. Wilber, J. A., Detection and Control of Hypertensive Disease in Georgia, U.S.A. Stamler, J., Stamler, R. and Pullman, T. N., Eds., *The Epidemiology of Hypertension,* Grune and Stratton, New York, N. Y., 439, 1967.

4. Wilber, J. A. and Barrow, J. G., Reducing Elevated Blood Pressure–Experience Found in a Community. *Minnesota Med., 52,* 1303, 1969.

5. Stamler, J., Schoenberger, J. A., Lindberg, H. A., Shekelle, R., Stoker, J. M., Epstein, M. B., deBoer, L., Stamler, R., Restivo, R., Gray, D. and Cain, W., Detection of Susceptibility to Coronary Disease. *Bull. N. Y. Acad. Med., 45,* 1306, 1969.

6. Inter-Society Commission for Heart Disease Resources. Hypertension Study Group. Guidelines for the Detection, Diagnosis, and Management of Hypertensive Populations. *Circulation, 44,* A623, 1971.

7. Schoenberger, J. A., Stamler, J. and Shekelle, R. B., *Current Status of Hypertension Control in an Industrial Population,* in press.

8. Veterans Administration Cooperative Study Group on Antihypertensive Agents. Effects of Treatment on Morbidity in Hypertension. II. Results in Patients with Diastolic Blood Pressure Averaging 90 through 114 mm Hg. *J. A. M. A., 213,* 1143, 1970.

9. Lew, E. A. and Seltzer, F., Use of the Life Table in Public Health. *Milbank Mem. Fund Quart., 48,* Suppl., 15, 1970.

10. Stamler, J., *Lectures on Preventive Cardiology,* Grune and Stratton, New York, N. Y., 1967.

11. National Diet-Heart Study Research Group. The National Diet-Heart Study Final Report. *Circulation, 33,* Suppl. 1, 1968.

12. Stamler, J., Acute Myocardial Infarction–Progress in Primary Prevention. *Brit. Heart J., 33,* (Suppl.) 145, 1971.

13. National Interagency Council on Smoking and Health. *World Conference on Smoking and Health*–A Summary of the Proceedings, Sept. 1967.

14. Cornfield, J., Joint Dependence of Risk of Coronary Heart Disease on Serum Cholesterol and Systolic Blood Pressure: A Discriminant Function Analysis. *Fed. Proc. 21,* 58, 1962.

Part I
Risk factors for ischemic heart disease

Chairman: *Lars Werkö*

Predicting coronary heart disease

By Ancel Keys

Collaborators

C. Aravanis, Athens, Greece
F. S. P. van Buchem, Haarlem, Netherlands
Henry Blackburn, Minneapolis, Minn., USA
R. Buzina, Zagreb, Yugoslavia
A. Carcondilas, Athens, Greece
B. S. Djordjevic, Belgrade, Yugoslavia
A. S. Dontas, Athens, Greece
F. Fidanza, Perugia, Italy
V. Josipovic, Belgrade, Yugoslavia
M. J. Karvonen, Helsinki, Finland
N. Kimura, Kurume, Japan
G. Lamm, Budapest, Hungary
D. Lekos, Athens, Greece
A. Menotti, Rome, Italy
I. Mohacek, Zagreb, Yugoslavia
M. Monti, Rome, Italy
S. Nedeljkovic, Belgrade, Yugoslavia
V. Puddu, Rome, Italy
Henry L. Taylor, Minneapolis, Minn., USA

The International Cooperative Study on Cardiovascular Epidemiology is concerned with some fourteen thousand men who were 40 through 59 years old at entry examination. Beginning in 1958, nineteen cohorts of men were enrolled in eight countries– Yugoslavia, the United States, Japan, Finland, Italy, the Netherlands, Greece and Hungary. Organization, methods, criteria, sampling and some entry characteristics of the men of thirteen cohorts in the Study were reported in 1967 in Acta Medica Scandinavica (1).

Here it is enough to stress the efforts to assure comparability of the diagnoses in the several cohorts–examinations conducted by international teams, exchange of personnel between examining teams, detailed instructions for procedure, standard forms for recording medical history and examination findings, central classification of all electrocardiograms, final diagnoses after review by Dr Henry Blackburn and Dr Alessandro Menotti on behalf of the coordination staff. To avoid possible bias between areas differing in availability and quality of medical care or records, second-hand reports without first-hand substantiation by our own staff were not accepted as diagnostic evidence.

In 1970 we reported some of the experience of five years of follow-up of men in seven countries; the findings in Hungary for the first five years were not then available so the publication, Monograph No. 29 of the American Heart Association, dealt with only seven countries (2).

The present report considers only six countries–Japan being omitted to eliminate possible differences related to race–and deals only with some new multivariate analyses. Most of this material is being reported elsewhere in somewhat more detail (3). The material for this purpose consists of data from five years of follow-up on over 11 000 men who were judged to be free of coronary heart disease at the entry examination. Coronary heart disease (CHD) is considered in two categories. First, death from CHD or definite myocardial infarction is here termed HARD CHD, not only because of the severity of the manifestation but also because "hard," meaning particularly rigorous, criteria are used for diagnosis. Second, there is CHD diagnosed with any criterion; ANY CHD includes HARD CHD, classical angina pectoris, and CHD diagnosis based on less specific clinical and electrocardiographic evidence for CHD.

Among these men who were judged to be free of CHD at the time of the entry examination, in five years 216 developed HARD CHD and a total of 615 men were judged to have developed ANY CHD. From this experience, utilizing the characteristics recorded for the men at the entry examination and the fact that some men developed CHD and most did not in the next five years, the effort was made to find useful predictors of the risk of becoming a "case" of CHD. Earlier, in this Cooperative Study and in other prospective studies such as that on business and professional men in Minnesota, started in 1947, and similar programs started later at Framingham, Massachusetts, and elsewhere, several single risk factors were identified–age, sex, serum cholesterol, blood pressure, smoking habit, etc (3).

But it is important to evaluate quantitatively the combined actions of such risk factors and to allow for possible confounding among the variables. One simple approach involves making broad classifications of each of the several variables, using cutting points of the measured variables to define "high" and "low," or "high," "medium" and "low," for blood pressure and for cholesterol and so on. Cross-classification then makes it possible to calculate the relative risk of men who are "high" in two risk factors as compared with men who are high in three or in only one, or are not high in any. From that simple method it seemed that the risk factors identified so far are additive, at least qualitatively. Such a method based on classes is, of course, only semi-quantitative and loses a great deal of information in the process of converting continuously distributed variables into discontinuous qualitative items. This method of cross-classification becomes hopelessly unwieldy when more than a very few variables are considered simultaneously (4). Obviously, a more powerful and more sophisticated multivariate approach is desirable. In the present analysis the main multivariate approach has been the use of multiple logistic equation:

(1) $\hat{y} = 1/[1 + e^{-(\alpha + \beta_1 x_1 + \beta_2 x_2 \ldots + \beta_k x_k)}]$,

in which e is the base of natural logarithms, 2.7183..., $\beta_1, \beta_2 \ldots \beta_k$ are coefficients for the corresponding variables $x_1, x_2 \ldots x_k$, e.g., age, systolic blood pressure, etc., while y is the probability that the individual characterized by values for $x_1, x_2 \ldots x_k$ will develop CHD.

Solution of the multiple logistic equation yields at discriminant function that best distinguishes cases from non-cases on the basis of the entry characteristics considered in the solution—age, blood pressure, and so on. Application of the coefficients to an individual's characteristics gives an estimate of the probability of an "event"—here the development of CHD—for that individual, the range being from zero, no chance at all, to one, certainty. For a group of individuals, the sum of their individual probabilities calculated in this way is an estimate or a prediction of the number of persons in the group who will be cases.

For most of the analyses reported here the multiple logistic equation has been solved by the method developed by Truett, Cornfield and Kannel (4). That method involves assumptions about the distribution of the variables in the "cases" and in "non-cases" that, in fact, are seldom fulfilled but, as will be seen, the results are solutions that are highly discriminatory and therefore of great practical utility. Another method of solving the multiple logistic equation, developed by Walker and Duncan (5), does not involve those assumptions but requires repeated computer runs to obtain successively converging approximations to coefficients that satisfy the criteria of maximum likelihood. The method of Walker and Duncan is superior in theory but is much more expensive in computer time. In parallel trials in the current study the method of Walker and Duncan could not be shown to produce any significantly better discimination than the method of Truett *et al* (4).

Coefficients obtained from some Walker-Duncan and Truett-Cornfield solutions of the multiple logistic equation are given in the Appendix of this report. Note that both methods provide estimated standard errors (SE) of the coefficients. The 95 per cent confidence limits of the coefficients are calculated as the coefficient ± 1.96 (SE).

In the present report the primary interest is in the utility of the discrimination or prediction achieved by the application of such coefficients to the individuals. Figure 1 shows 78 cases of HARD CHD distributed into deciles of the array of values of probability estimated from five entry characteristics: age, systolic blood pressure, serum cholesterol concentration, smoking habit and body mass index. Body mass index, a measure of relative body weight, is calculated as the body weight, in kg, divided by

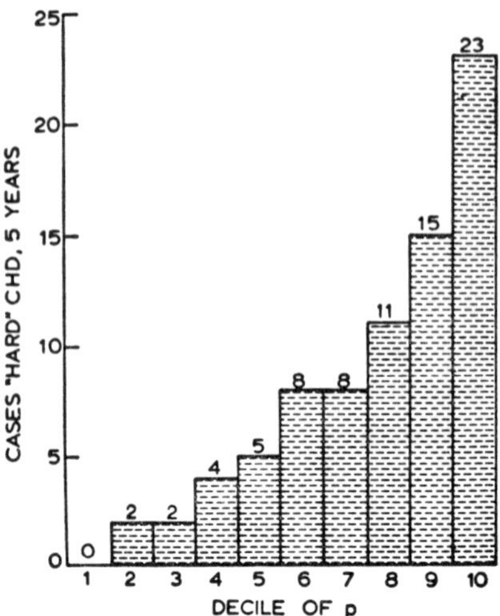

Fig. 1. CHD deaths and infarctions (HARD CHD, N = 78) observed in 5 years among 2 404 U.S. railroad men, aged 40–59 and CHD-free at the start, arranged in decile classes of probability of HARD CHD calculated from coefficients found by solving the multiple logistic equation for the variables of age, systolic blood pressure, serum cholesterol concentration, smoking habit and body mass index using the entry data on these men.

the square of the height (body length) in meters. Among 240 men at risk in the bottom decile of estimated probability, none developed HARD CHD; among an equal number of men in the top decile, 23 developed HARD CHD. Among 481 men classified from their entry characteristics as being in the top 20 per cent in estimated risk, 38 died from CHD or had a definite infarction in five years, the corresponding number for the bottom 20 per cent being only 2 men. The observed incidence was 19 times greater in the top than in the bottom quintile.

Figure 2 shows the distribution of the 210 U.S. railroad men who were given a diagnosis of ANY CHD during five years of follow-up. The discrimination is somewhat inferior to that achieved when only HARD CHD was considered but the risk ratio of cases in the top compared with cases in the bottom quintile is still impressive: 85 vs. 13 or a risk ratio of 6.5 to one.

The corresponding analysis of the five-year experience versus entry characteristics for HARD CHD among 8 728 European mean, CHD-free at entry, is summarized in Figure 3. In the top decile of the distribution of estimated probability of developing HARD CHD, 46 men actually developed HARD CHD; among an equal number of men at risk in the bottom decile, only two men became patients with HARD CHD.

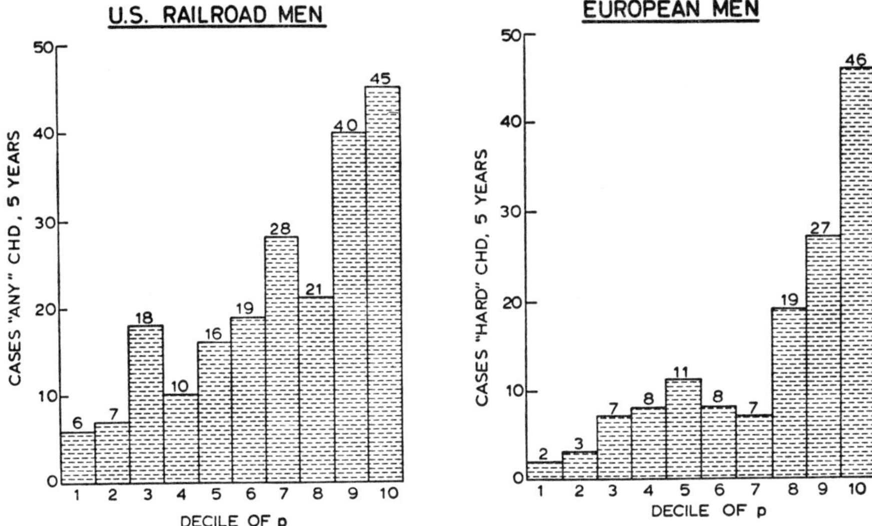

Fig. 2. Same as Figure 1 but for all diagnoses of CHD (ANY CHD, N=210) in the 5-year follow-up of those U.S. men.

Fig. 3. CHD deaths and infactions (HARD CHD, N=138) observed in 5 years among 8 728 European men aged 40–59 and CHD-free at the start. Same as Figure 1 but using data and multiple logistic equation coefficients for these European men.

Figure 4 summarizes the corresponding findings for five-year incidence of ANY CHD diagnosis–405 men–among the same 8 728 Europeans. Without the information provided from the analysis with the data on age, blood pressure, serum cholesterol, smoking habit and body mass index, the expectation would be 40.5 cases in each of the classes of 873 men in the top

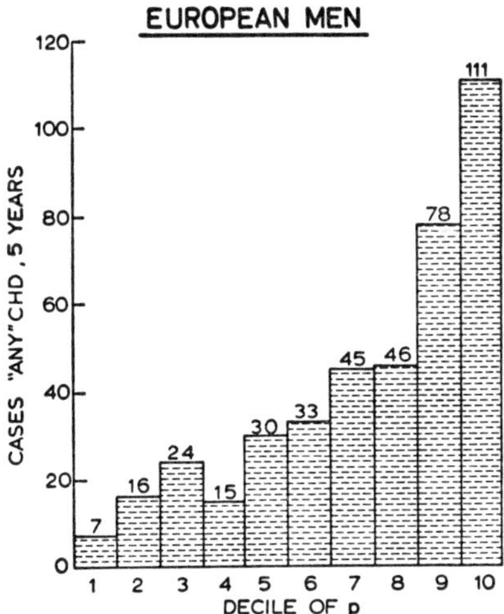

Fig. 4. Same as Figure 3 but for all CHD diagnoses (ANY CHD, N=405) in the follow-up of those European men.

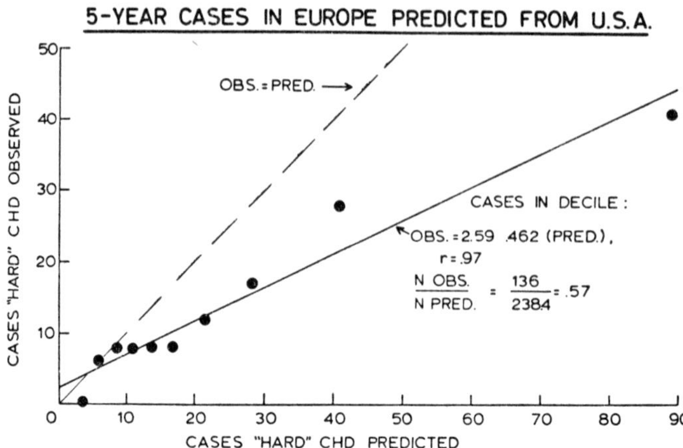

Fig. 5. Cases of HARD CHD in 5 years in the European men in decile classes of probability predicted by applying the USA multiple logistic equation coefficients to the variables as measured in the European men.

and in the bottom decile. Figure 4 shows that from this present analysis the top decile provided 111/7 = 15.9 times more cases of CHD than did the bottom decile.

Such results indicate the power of this multivariate analysis but a crucial question concerns *prediction*: how well can CHD in one population be predicted from findings on another population? Figure 5 shows the result of predicting HARD CHD in the European men from the solution of the multiple logistic equation using U.S. railroad experience. The *relative* prediction is good, the correlation between observed and expected numbers of cases in the decile classes being r = .97. Thirty per cent of the observed cases of HARD CHD were concentrated in the top 10 per cent of

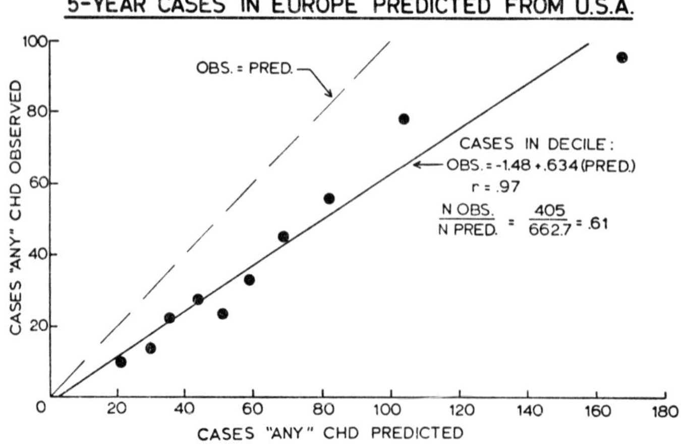

Fig. 6. Same as Figure 5 but for cases of ANY CHD in the 5-year follow-up.

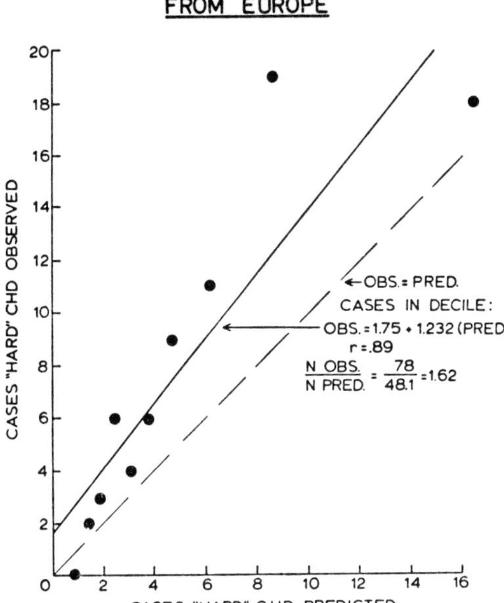

Fig. 7. Cases of HARD CHD in 5 years in the American men in the decile classes of probability predicted by applying the European multiple logistic equation coefficients to the variables as measured in the American men.

the probability distribution while no cases occurred in the bottom 10 per cent of that distribution. Absolutely, however, there is a great discrepancy. From the same number of men in the U.S. with identical characteristics of age, blood pressure, serum cholesterol, smoking habit and body mass index, the expectation would be 238.4 instead of the 136 cases of HARD CHD observed. The incidence among the European men was only 57 per cent of the expectation to match the U.S. railroad men.

Figure 6 shows that almost the same relationship holds when ANY CHD is considered. The coefficient of correlation between the numbers of men predicted from U.S. experience and those observed in Europe in deciles of probability is =.97; in the top decile, 97 cases occurred, only ten cases were found in the bottom decile. But again the absolute numbers are greatly discrepant; 662.7 total cases predicted but only 405, or 61 per cent observed.

The converse predictions, CHD being predicted for the U.S. railroad men from the experience in Europe, are summarized in Figures 7 and 8. The *relative* risk of men classified within the U.S. group is well predicted. For HARD CHD the coefficient of correlation between numbers expected and numbers observed in the decile classes of probability is r=.89; for

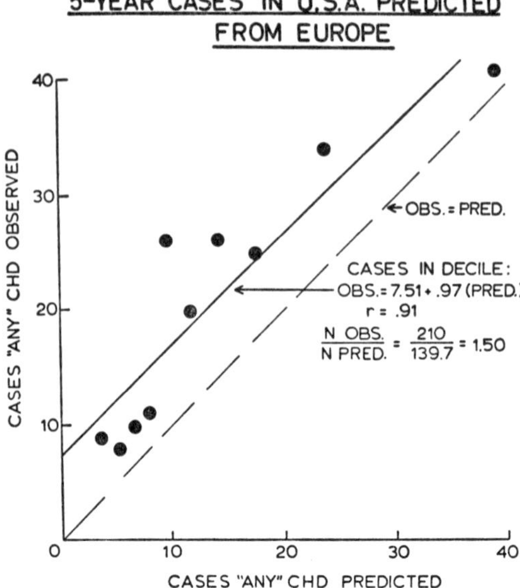

Fig. 8. Same as Figure 7 but for cases of ANY CHD in the 5-year follow-up.

ANY CHD the figure is r =.91. For HARD CHD the equation solved for Europe discriminated top and bottom quintile classes which proved to provide 37 and two cases, respectively, a ratio of 18.5 to one. But in total numbers of cases the incidence among the U.S. railroad men was grossly excessive–62 per cent excessive for HARD CHD, 50 per cent for ANY CHD.

Follow-up studies very similar to the International Cooperative Study have been in progress for some years in Framingham, Mass., in Albany, N.Y., and in Chicago (two studies). Combined into what may be termed the "»-POOL," these follow-up studies cover 6 221 men aged 40–59 and considered to be CHD-free at entry. During five years of follow-up and re-examination, 223 men in the 4-POOL were reported to have developed HARD CHD. Drs W. B. Kannel, J. T. Doyle, Jeremiah Stamler and Oglesby Paul kindly allowed the test with their data of multiple logistic solutions from the U.S. railroad and European experience in the International Cooperative Study.

Figure 9 compares numbers of cases of HARD CHD observed and predicted from the multiple logistic equation solved with data from the U.S. railroad men. The 4-POOL relative prediction is good, with r =.95, but in absolute numbers the 4-POOL CHD cases were excessive by about 41 per cent. Part of that discrepancy may reflect CHD cases found at interim examinations which would have been missed with only a single five-year

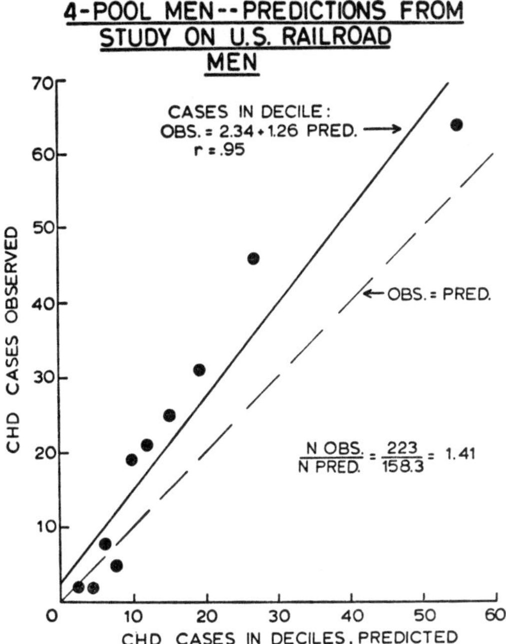

Fig. 9. HARD CHD in 5 years among the 4-POOL men as observed and as predicted from data on age, systolic blood pressure, serum cholesterol, smoking habit and body mass index using coefficients in the multiple logistic equation for U.S. railroad men.

re-examination, as in the International Cooperative Study, or which we would not have accepted as cases because only secondhand diagnostic evidence was available. In the 4-POOL studies two or more re-examinations in five years tended to be the rule and second-hand evidence from hospital records and from other physicians was utilized for diagnoses.

But such explanations could not remove the huge discrepancy shown in Figure 10. The 4-POOL men had more than double the incidence of CHD that would be expected from experience with European men matched in these five characteristics. In the 4-POOL, 223 men developed HARD CHD; for Europeans of the same age, blood pressure, serum cholesterol, smoking habit and body mass index, the expectation would be only 104 men. Compared with the European men, the 4-POOL men were more than twice as susceptible to CHD.

Analyses including other entry characteristics do not remove the conclusion of a grossly excessive CHD frequency, compared to men in Europe, among the American men—railroad men as well as 4-POOL men. Relative body weight, body fatness, physical activity have been incorporated in multiple logistic solutions and they fail to explain the difference in CHD

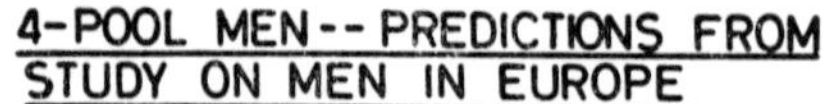

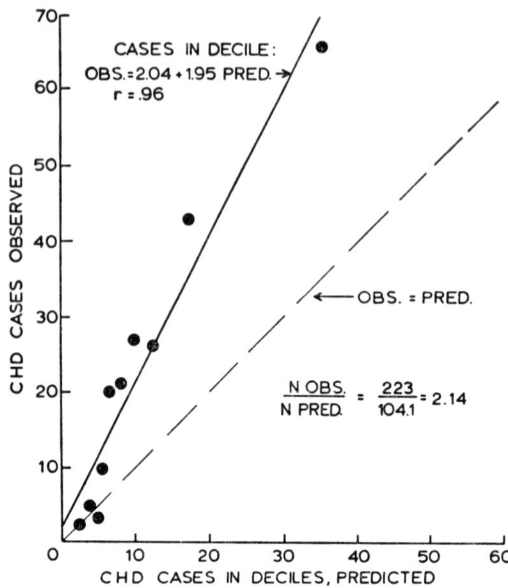

Fig. 10. Same as Figure 9 but cases of HARD CHD in the 4-POOL as predicted from coefficients in the multiple logistic equation obtained from data on men in Europe.

incidence. In fact, in the multivariate analysis those variables did not prove to be risk factors at all; the coefficients obtained for them in the solution of the multiple logistic equation have such large standard errors as to be statistically not significantly different from zero. And when those variables and their coefficients are included in the analysis there is no improvement in discrimination or prediction over the analysis omitting them.

Discussion

The multiple logistic equation has proved to be exceedingly useful in the multivariate analyses of the data from the International Cooperative Study on Cardiovascular Epidemiology. Mathematically, the equation has advantages and the method of Truett and Cornfield provides a convenient method of solution without great demand for computer power and time. But there is no theoretical reason why other models might not do as well or even better in describing the multivariate situation. The more common and familiar multiple regression equation has also been applied to the current data. That equation is:

(2) $y=a+b_1x_1+b_2x_2...b_kx_k$;

the coefficients $b_1,b_2...b_k$ are simply multiplied by the values of the corresponding variables $x_1,x_2...x_k$, and the results are added to the constant, a, to yield an estimate of y, the dependent variable. Here, y can be considered as a measure of the amount of CHD and equation 2) can be applied to the question of discrimination in the same way as the multiple logistic has been applied in this report. From the solution to equation 2), values of y can be calculated for each of the individuals, those values can then be arrayed and the men distributed into deciles or other fractiles of the array of y values.

In terms of discriminating power with the present material, the multiple regression model proved to be no less powerful than the multiple logistic. At least, no test so far applied to comparisons of results with two approaches shows any significant difference.

Multiple logistic solutions using entry data on age, systolic pressure, serum cholesterol and smoking habit have great and universal value in predicting the relative risk of developing coronary heart disease among middle-aged white men. The prediction is not improved by considering relative weight, body fatness, diastolic pressure or physical activity as additional variables. It is concluded that other variables besides those considered here must be important in the etiology.

References

1. Keys, A., Aravanis, C., Blackburn, H., van Buchem, F. S. P., Buzina, R., Djordjevic, B. S., Dontas, A. S., Fidanza, F., Karvonen, M. J., Kimura, N., Lekos, D., Monti, M., Puddu, V., Taylor, H. L.: Epidemiological studies related to coronary heart disease of men aged 40–59 in seven countries. *Acta Med. Scand.,* Suppl. 460, 1967.
2. Keys, A. (ed.): Coronary heart disease in seven countries. *Amer. Heart Assoc. Monograph,* No. 29, 1970. Also *Circulation,* Suppl. 1, vols. 41, 42, 1970.
3. Keys, A., Aravanis, C., Blackburn, H., van Buchem, F. S. P., Buzina, R., Djordjevic, B. S., Fidanza, F., Karvonen, M., Menotti, A., Puddu, V., Taylor, H. L. The probability of middle-aged men developing coronary heart disease in five years. *Circulation* 45:815, 1972.
4. Truett, J., J. Cornfield, W. Kannel: Multivariate analysis of the risk of coronary heart disease. *J. Chronic Dis. 20:* 511, 1967.
5. Walker, S. H., Duncan D. B.: Estimation of the probability of an event as a function of several independent variables. *Biometrica 54:* 167, 1967.

Acknowledgements

Full acknowledgement of financial support and of the help of the many individuals and organizations that made possible the data reported here is given in previous publications, notably Supplementum No. 460 of Acta medica Scandinavica in 1967 (1) and American Heart Association Monograph No. 29 in 1970 (2). It is proper here, however, to express gratitude to the U.S. Public Health Service National Heart and Lung Institute for providing the initial funds (grant No. 04697 to A.K.) and the majority of subsequent financial support.

Appendix

Coefficients, and the constant alpha, from solution of the multiple logistic equation using data on 5-year CHD incidence and entry characteristics for men aged 40–59 and CHD-free at entry. T–C and W–D are, respectively, solutions with methods of Truett, Cornfield and Kannel (3) and of Walker and Duncan (4). Values in ( ) are estimated standard errors of the coefficients.

	Any CHD				Hard CHD			
	U.S. railroad		Europe		U.S. railroad		Europe	
	W–D	T–C	W–D	T–C	W–D	T–C	W–D	T–C
The constant alpha	−8.6337	−8.9683	−11.0754	−11.3664	−13.1677	−13.0228	−12.8620	−13.1783
Age in years	.0327 (.0147)	.0315 (.0145)	.0714 (.0103)	.0653 (.0097)	.0817 (.0242)	.0696 (.0230)	.0812 (.0173)	.0728 (.0165)
Systolic BP, mm Hg	.0163 (.0036)	.0192 (.0041)	.0145 (.0023)	.0177 (.0027)	.0151 (.0055)	.0181 (.0064)	.0154 (.0036)	.0193 (.0045)
Serum cholesterol, mg/dl	.0053 (.0017)	.0052 (.0018)	.0074 (.0009)	.0082 (.0010)	.0089 (.0026)	.0094 (.0028)	.0087 (.0014)	.0102 (.0017)
Physical activity[a]	−.1985 (.1692)	−.1989 (.1659)	.0924 (.0584)	.0805 (.0589)	−.2432 (.2793)	−.2666 (.2616)	−.0635 (.0954)	−.0905 (.1001)
Sum skin-folds, mm	.0090 (.0065)	.0088 (.0067)	.0084 (.0048)	.0076 (.0050)	.0086 (.0103)	.0077 (.0105)	.0007 (.0081)	−.0014 (.0085)
Smoking habit[b]	.1933 (.0478)	.1928 (.0462)	.0647 (.0312)	.0639 (.0308)	.2406 (.0764)	.2382 (.0729)	.1099 (.0515)	.1000 (.0524)

[a] In habitual occupation graded as 1 = sedentary, 2 = moderately active, 3 = very active or heavy physical work.
[b] 3 = non smoker, 4 = <5 cigarettes/day, 5 = 5–9 per day, 6 = 10–19 per day, 7 = 20–29 per day, 8 = 30 or more cigarettes per day.

Risk factors for developing myocardial infarction and other diseases. The "Men born in 1913" study

By Gösta Tibblin

On the official (WHO) ranking list of age-specific death rates for cardiovascular diseases (CVD) Sweden is rather far down the scale (6). But if we consider the major causes of death the same diseases dominate the picture. Among men at age 50–54, 40 per cent of the deaths are due to cardiocascular diseases (CVD) and at age 70–74 years the same figure is 60 per cent. The mortality and morbidity in CVD is thus a major problem also in Sweden thought the favourable position on the ranking list (6).

One way of improving our knowledge about the etiology and natural history of myocardial infaction is to perform a prospective population study. This approach allows identification of risk factors which can be used to construct hypotheses and may give guidelines for preventive intervention studies which, if positive, can support different hypotheses constructed. This does not mean that the risk factors identified also have to be causative agents.

In various prospective studies a large number of risk factors has been identified. In order to construct hypotheses regarding etiology and therapy it is necessary to evaluate the influence of each of the single variables when the other variables are kept constant. The only risk factor which by all investigators is regarded as always present is age. Keys and coworker have shown how the incidence in ischemic heart diseases (IHD-deaths and myocardial infarctions) is not far from being linear in a semilogarithmic plot. (1). Most studies have limited the number of investigated men to below around 5 000, many only around 1 000. Because of the rather low incidence per year it has not been possible to divide the study group in groups with more uniform age. The results have thus at best been presented in age-groups at the start of the study comprising ages 30–59, 40–59 and sometimes 40–49 and 50–59. This necessarily obscures the results especially as the age distribution within these groups does not have to be uniform.

There is another reason for the advisability of eliminating age in such studies. Almost all risk factors are by themselves related to age. This means that all studies of age–heterogenous series tend to get skewed regarding the relative importance of individual risk factors and may for example underestimate the influence of smoking while overemphasizing other factors.

The present report is a part of a long term study attempting to investigate the development of myocardial infarction in a series selected so as to avoid the influence of the agefactor. All the participants are men born the same year–1913 and living in Göteborg, Sweden.

This report will concentrate on a circumscribed questions; Are the usual "risk factors" specific for the development of myocardial infarction? Or are the common "risk factors" also precursors of other diseases, identifying individuals or groups with high overall morbidity and mortality?

Method

Göteborg on the west-coast of Sweden is an industrial city with near half a million inhabitants. It has one hospital only taking care of all acute diseases. An accurate population register checked yearly and a stable population offers us an unique opportunity to study the natural history of chronic disease in particular cardiovascular diseases. The "Men born in 1913 study" has been in continous operation since 1963 when the first crossectional study was performed. The derivation and composition of the population under study has been described previously in detail (4). An analysis of the small non-participation group has also been done (3). Of the originally 973 subjects selected for study, 855 were investigated at the Sahlgren' hospital (the participation group) and 40 were studied at their home (originally not willing to participate). In 1967 a follow-up study was done. In this follow-up 803 subjects of the 855 took part. In 1968 a randomly selected subsample of the men born in 1913 was studied concerning body build.

In 1970 a postal questionnaire was sent out in order to get information about the development of cardiovascular disease in the group. The next clinical follow-up is planned to occur in 1973. Through a myocardial infarction register established since 1968 in Göteborg it has been possible to continuously identify all new cases of clinical myocardial infarction and sudden death in the community.

In 1963 and in 1967 all subjects were examined in the out-patient clinic of Medical clinic I, Sahlgren's hospital. A detailed history and physical examination were completed by physicians assigned to the study. Questionnaires recommended by WHO have been used for defining angina pectoris, chronic bronchitis, infarction pain and breathlessness.

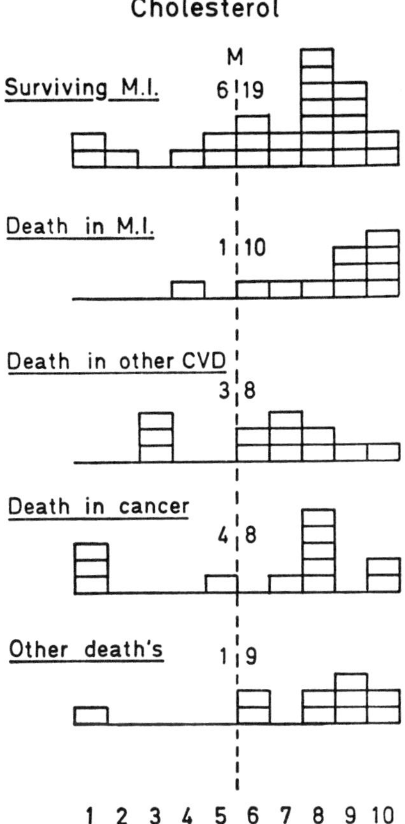

Fig. 1. Number of patients with different diseases in deciles of cholesterol.

Criteria for myocardial infarction

Criteria used for myocardial infaction was hospitalization with a clinical diagnoses of myocardial infarction, or fresh myocardial infarction at autopsy. The clinical and pathological diagnosis were established by the responsible clinicians and pathologists resp. actively in all cases. In the crossectional study in 1963 a clinical diagnoses of myocardial infarction with remaining ECG evidence were also accepted even without previous hospitalization. In one case positive evidence from coronary angiography was accepted as proof of a previous myocardial infarction.

Results

Prevalence. In 1963, 12 men fullfilled the criteria of myocardial infarction. The prevalence rate (cases per 100 000) is 140. It was possible to obtain death certificates from the Central Bureau of Statistics for all male sub-

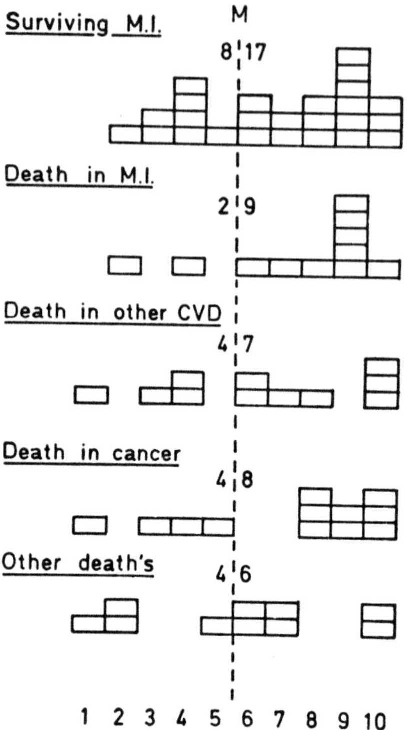

Fig. 2. Number of patients with different diseases in deciles of triglycerides.

jects born in 1913 on the same day as the selected subjects in the present study and registered as dying in Göteborg between 1950–1962. During this period out of 33 death's three died of myocardial infaction. In the non-participation group there was one case of clinical myocardial infarction. This means that of 1 006 men (973 in the study sample and 33 death's before 1963) 16 developed myocardial infarction before 50 years of age.

Incidence

Of the eleven cases of fresh myocardial infarction deaths who occured during close to eight years two cases had myocardial infaction already before the initial examination 1963 and were thus not CHD free at that time. From 1963 to 1 of Nov. 1971 further 25 new subjects developed myocardial infarction, were hospitalized and have survived up to now. The annual incidence of M.I. in this 50 year old cohort can be calculated to

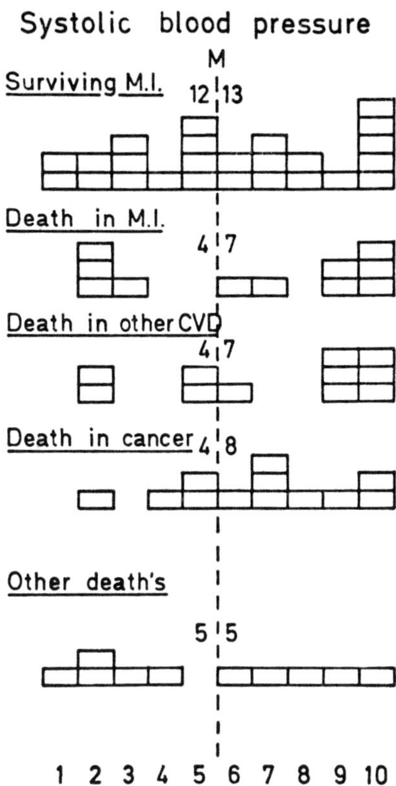

Fig. 3. Number of patients with different diseases in deciles of blood pressure.

5.2 per 1 000 and year of the 843 M.I.-free men examined in 1963 between the ages of 50 and 58.

Up to now 33 non-myocardial infarction deaths have occurred. In the further analysis they have been used as comparison groups in order to ascertain the specificity of the most conventional risk factors' for myocardial infarction.

The autopsy rate is high (42/44). One subject dying in a traffic accident and one case of sudden death were not autopsied. Sudden death is often defined as witnessed unexpected death occurring within a short time span-minutes or hours. This mode of death has been regarded as a manifestation of coronary disease. Because of the high autopsy rate in Göteborg it has been possible to identify a series of subjects experiencing sudden death without anatomical evidence of fresh myocardial infarction. They have been compared with another group dying suddenly and at autopsy showing fresh myocardial infarction. The numbers in the two groups are small (7 and 11) but the difference between the two groups regarding the num-

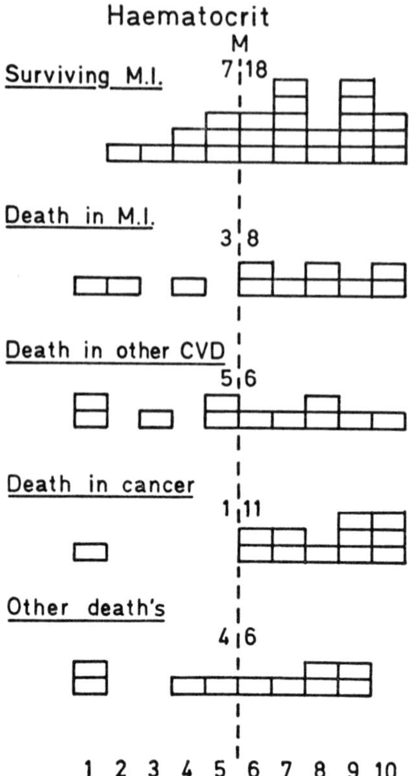

Fig. 4. Number of patients with different diseases in deciles of haematocrit.

bers extent of risk factors registered in 1963 is striking. The only factor which was common in the two groups was alcohol problems. The other risk factors, cigarette smoking, serumcholesterol, triglycerides, heart volume and haematocrit occured infrequently in the sudden death group without myocardial infarction.

The lack of evidence of fresh myocardial infarction at autopsy does not justify that individuals with this type of sudden death and patients dying suddenly with myocardial infarction are treated together as one homogenous group. There may also be several reasons to doubt whether sudden death has the same etiological background as other manifestations of coronary heart disease. In this study sudden death without signs of fresh myocardial infarction is grouped as other CVD.

Risk factors

All patients with myocardial infarction surviving M.I. and death in M.I. are presented in relation to values for risk factors in 1963 divided in

Table 1. Incidiences of different disease categories among subjects with alcohol problems and being smokers.

	Alcohol problems ($n = 179$)	No alcohol problems ($n = 676$)	Smoking ($n = 480$)	No smoking ($n = 375$)
Surviving M.I.	5.6	2.2	5.0	0.3
† M.I.	3.4	0.7	1.9	0.5
† other C.V.D.	2.2	1.0	1.3	1.3
† cancer	1.7	1.3	2.1	0.5
Other death's	2.8	0.7	1.7	0.5

quintiles for serum-cholesterol, triglycerides, haematocrit and systolic blood pressure. This relation is compared to the 33 patients dying of other reasons grouped in relation to the same risk factors values of 1963. These 33 subjects were classified as healthy in 1963. In Fig. 1–4 it is demonstrated that the risk factors seems thus to be related both to the later development of myocardial infarction and to death of other causes.

In Table 1 the same relation to two further risk factors are presented. Both tobacco smoking and the existence of social alcohol problems bear a similar relation to myocardial infarction and other causes of death.

In order to compare the strength of the relationships between different risk factors and different disease categories the ratio of cases above and below the median of the serum cholesterol, triglycerides, systolic blood pressure and haematocrit has been used. Concerning alcohol problems and smoking the ratio of incidence was used.

The five disease categories were also ranked. From Table 2 it is clear that the ratio in all cases is 1 or more. It means that there is at least a trend these risk factors are actual for all disease categories. Death in M.I. has the lowest ranking sum (10–11). Of interest is that M.I. survivers and death in cancer is very close to each other (16 respectively 17).

Discussion

In the present study 16 men out of 1 006 have developed myocardial infarction before 50 years of age. The annual incidence of myocardial infarction after 50 years of age up to about age 58 is 5.2 per 1 000 per year. This compares to an age-standardized average yearly infarct incidence rates per 1 000 men aged 40–59 of 6.5 in U.S. Railroad men and 5.7 in rural districts of Finland (1). This study differs from other population studies of CHD in the following ways:

Table 2. Ranking order of different disease categories concerning risk factors.

	Chol.		Trigl.		S. B. P.		Haematocr.		Alcohol problems		Smoking	
	Ratio > M/ < M	Ranking order	Ratio > M/ < M	Ranking order	Ratio > M/ < M	Rankign order	Ratio > M/ < M	Ranking order	Ratio	Ranking order	Ratio	Ranking order
M.I. Survivors	3.2	3	2.1	2	1.1	4	2.6	3	2.6	3	16.7	1
Death in M.I.	10.0	1	4.5	1	1.8	2–3	2.7	2	4.9	1	3.8	3
Death in other CVD	2.7	4	1.8	4	1.8	2–3	1.2	5	2.2	4	1.0	5
Death in cancer	2.0	5	2.0	3	2.0	1	11.0	1	1.3	5	4.2	2
Other death's	9.0	2	1.5	5	1.0	5	1.5	4	4.0	2	3.4	45

1. The target population is from an urban area in a country with low incidence of deaths in myocardial infarction at early ages.
2. Care has been taken to define and select a representative cohort for study.
3. Regarding coronary heart disease only clinical cases—living or dead—with M.I. have been included.

The criteria used for myocardial infarction was a firm hospital diagnosis or clear cut pathological evidence at post-mortem of fresh myocardial infarction. The autopsy frequency was high (42/44) allowing a proper subgrouping of cases. Without autopsy the value of death certificates is limited.

When age is properly taken into consideration—all men were born the same year—the well-known risk factors for developing myocardial infarction as serum cholesterol, triglycerides and tobacco smoking were still operating. Some risk factors seem also to be of importance in this population that is haematocrit and social alcohol problems.

Systolic blood pressure was also related to the development of myocardial infarction. This influence has, however, been interfered with an anti-hypertensive treatment (5).

In order to investigate how specific the mention risk factors are for myocardial infarction other groups were studied for comparison—all cases dying from different causes were grouped in four categories. It was found that the occurrence of risk factors increased the likelihood of early death from whatever cause. In this context it is of interest that in the U S National Pooling Project, comprising 7 342 white males age 30–59 at entry the ageadjusted 10-years death rate in those with three risk factors was 82/1000 men in CHD, 65/1000 men in other disease than CHD, while for those with no risk factor, the same figures were 13 and 17 respectively. The relation was similar when calculated for groups with one or two risk factors only (2).

These data made it rather obvious that most of the risk factors that has earlier been considered to be rather specific for the later occurence of myocardial infarction on the contrary may lack specificity and seem to be almost as valid for later death.

How can the predictive value of risk factors such as serumcholesterol, triglycerides, tobacco-smoking and haemotocrit for later non-myocardial death be explained? It may be that all these factors are agents facilitating the development of many serious diseases, something which is known for tobacco-smoking. The importance of these and other factors in this regard can only be elucidated through prospective intervention studies.

Such an intervention trial is under way in similar age groups in Göteborg. If measures aimed at the known risk factors will prove to be effective on the future development of disease there should be a drop not only in the incidence of M.I. but also in deaths from all causes if these factors are in any way causative, and not only predictive. Results from this study will be forthcoming toward the middle of the 1970's.

Another explanations of the findings in the present study is that behind the "risk factors" one or several other more strictly causative factors are operating. Variables such as personality traits, behavioural or social circumstances have been discussed and also studied in a limited way. Behind the habit of tobacco-smoking, high serum-lipids and other risk factors some common factor such as for example behaviour type A or serious life changes may be causative or add substantially to the overall risk.

This background factor may be a more obvious link to all kind of premature death, such as rapid aging. Of risk factors discussed in this study all except smoking and haematocrit increase by age. In the studied group premature aging might be responsible for the co-existence of both an increased number of risk factors and the development of myocardial infarction and death of non-cardiovascular cause.

An attempt to test this hypothesis is to compare patients in the middle 50's with myocardial infarction and age-matched patients with other serious diseases such as malignant tumors in an early stage and establish wheather they have more signs of aging than controls concerning skin elasticity, grayness of the hair, memory, renal funktion, hearing, vision etc.

If so, variables of aging should be studied in a prospective way in order to define other indices for the later development of serious diseases. This might then lead to better possibilities for overall preventive medicine.

The present results make it difficult to support a single factor hypothesis for the development of myocardial infarction. It is also hard to construct a multifactorial hypothesis which can explain both the development of myocardial infarction and other premature death.

The question of the cause of myocardial infarction needs a fresh look including a better analysis of the old and possible addition of some new risk factors.

The multifactorial hypothesis for the development of myocardial infarction should also take into consideration the possibility that some risk factors–perhaps mostly biochemical or metabolicpromote or indicate the development of vascular disease, while others–such as psycho-social, or sudden severe life changes–may act close to the acute catastrophe of myocardial infarction and precipitate the acute event in a vulnerable individual.

Summary

In a prospective population study of 855 men born in the same year and followed 7 and a half year several risk factors were found for the development of fresh myocardial infarction. All these risk factors were also related to the development of non-cardiovascular deaths.

References

1. Key, A.: Coronary Heart Disease in Seven Countries. *American Heart Association Monograph,* No. 29, 1970.
2. Report of Inter-Society Commission for Heart Disease Resources. *Circulation 42,* July 1970.
3. Tibblin, G.: A population study of 50-year-old men–an analysis of the non-participation group. *Acta Med. Scand. 178:* 453, 1965.
4. Tibblin, G.: High blood pressure in men aged 50. *Acta Med. Scand.,* Suppl. 470, 1967.
5. Tibblin, G. & Bengtsson, C.: Detection and treatment of hypertension in a community. *Milbank Memorial Fund Quaterly 47:* 160, 1969.
6. Vedin, A., Wilhelmsson, C., Bolander, A.-M. & Werkö, L.: Mortality trends in Sweden 1951–1968 with special reference to cardiovascular causes of death. *Acta Med. Scand.* Suppl. 515, 1970.

The National Cooperative Pooling Project in the United States

By Jeremiah Stamler

Nature and Purpose of the Pooling Project

The Pooling Project in the United States is a national cooperative effort under the aegis of the Council of Epidemiology of the American Heart Association. It involves eight long-term prospective studies of adult cardiovascular disease (1, la.–lm.).*

The main objective of the Pooling Project is to take advantage of the greater numbers available from the combined data of several similar studies, in order to accomplish analyses of greater precision and refinement than is possible in any one study.

The principal concern is with the relationship between several traits, habits and medical findings recorded at initial examination and subsequent risk of experiencing cardiovascular events, non-fatal and fatal, over the ensuing decade in white males free at entry of evidence of coronary heart disease (CHD).

Prerequisites for Pooling Data from Different Studies

At least four prerequisites had to be met for success in this effort to pool data from these several prospective studies of adult cardiovascular disease that had been designed and carried out more or less independently:

1. They had to be generally similar in their design, measurements made at initial examination and methods of measurement.

---

* These studies and their Principal Investigators are: Albany Civil Servants Study–Joseph T. Doyle; Chicago Peoples Gas Company Study–Jeremiah Stamler, David M. Berkson and Howard A. Lindberg; Chicago Western Electric Company Study–Oglesby Paul; Framingham Community Study–Thomas R. Dawber and William B. Kannel; Los Angeles Civil Servants Study–John M. Chapman; Minneapolis-St. Paul Business and Professional Men Study–Ancel Keys, Henry L. Taylor and Henry Blackburn; Tecumseh Community Study–Frederick H. Epstein; U.S. Railroad Men Study–Henry L. Taylor, Henry Blackburn and Ancel Keys.

This effort is being coordinated by Professors Frederick H. Epstein and Felix Moore at the University of Michigan School of Public Health in Ann Arbor, Michigan.

At the present time, final tabulations of the pooled data from the eight studies are being completed, and a final report is being written. Preliminary data are available from a set of special tabulations done during the summer of 1970 for reports to the World Cardiological Congress in London and for the Report on the Primary Prevention of the Atherosclerotic Diseases of the Inter-Society Commission on Heart Disease Resources (l, 1a.–1m., 2). These data are the subject of this presentation. They encompass findings on 7 342 white men age 30–59 at initial examination–pooled data then available from five of the cooperating studies.

2. Their populations had to manifest a generally similar distribution of the risk factors under investigation.
3. The studies had to record generally similar rates for the key cardiovascular disease end points.
4. The relationship between risk factors and cardiovascular events had to be generally similar among the studies.

For the last three of these four prerequisites for data pooling, it is possible to apply statistical tests to assess whether the preconditions have been met, and this is of course being done. However, the term *similar* in the above propositions cannot be defined in purely statistical terms, but rather —as is almost always the case—must ultimately rely upon the joint judgement of the investigators. The preliminary data of this report, from a pool of five studies, are deemed to be "poolable".

Preliminary Findings of the Pooling Project

In Figures 1–3, separate analyses are presented on three factors—cholesterolemia, blood pressure, and cigarette smoking status at initial examination and age-adjusted 10-year incidence rates for four end points. As is evident, risk of developing premature coronary heart disease (CHD)—including sudden death and all fatal CHD—is related to serum cholesterol level (Fig. 1) (2). Since CHD is the single most important cause of death for white Americans of this age, mortality from all causes is also related to cholesterolemia. For first major coronary events (nonfatal and fatal myocardial infaction, plus sudden death attributed to CHD), there is an almost fourfold greater risk for those at the upper end of the distribution (i.e., above 299 mg./dl.) compared to those at the lower end (i.e., below 175). Almost half of the new events—296 of 596—occurred among the third of the men with levels of 250 or above. This upper third had a 10-year CHD risk about twice that of the rest of the population (119 per 1 000 vs. 61).

The findings for blood pressure and these same end points are similar (Fig. 2) (2). While Figure 2 deals only with diastolic pressure, essentially the same results are available for systolic pressure. Compared to optimal levels of blood pressure, even "modest" elevations (i.e., diastolics of 85–94 or 95–104 mm. Hg) are associated with grossly higher risks—a point of great practical significance for clinicians.

To put this important observation in a more general way, for each of these quantitative variables, there is a steady increment in risk as level of the variable rises. As cholesterol concentration—or blood pressure—increases, risk increases. The relationships are continuous. There is no evidence of

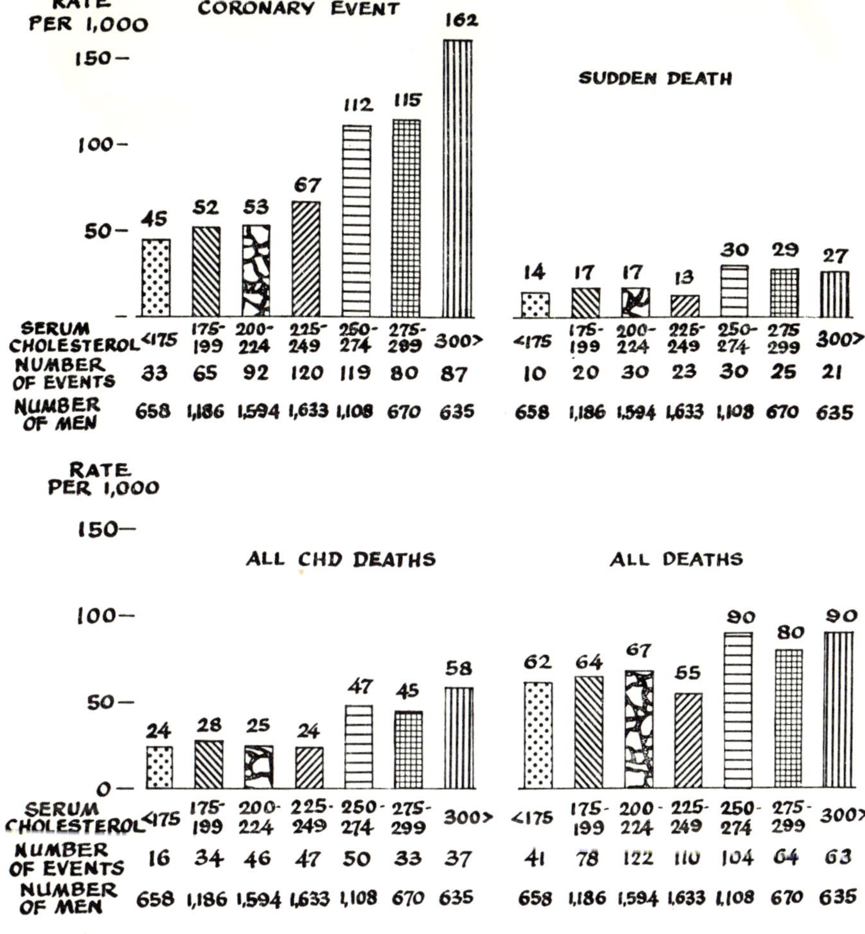

Fig. 1. National Cooperative Pooling Project; serum cholesterol level at entry and 10-year age-adjusted rates per 1 000 men for: first any major coronary event, sudden death (upper graph), and coronary death, death from all causes (lower Graph); first major coronary event includes nonfatal MI, fatal MI, sudden death due to CHD; U.S. white males age 30–59 at entry; all rates age-adjusted by 10-year age groups to the U.S. white male population, 1960 (1, la.–m., 2).

a critical level which divides "normal" subgroups (i.e., subgroups "immune" to premature coronary heart disease) from CHD-prone "abnormal" subgroups. For individuals, this conclusion from the massive epidemiologic data can be reformulated as follows: The higher the risk factor level, the greater the probability of developing coronary disease. This is important from the point of view of instituting preventive measures. The greater the probability, the greater the need for prophylaxis—but there is no single "screening level" separating those in need of prophylaxis from those who are not.

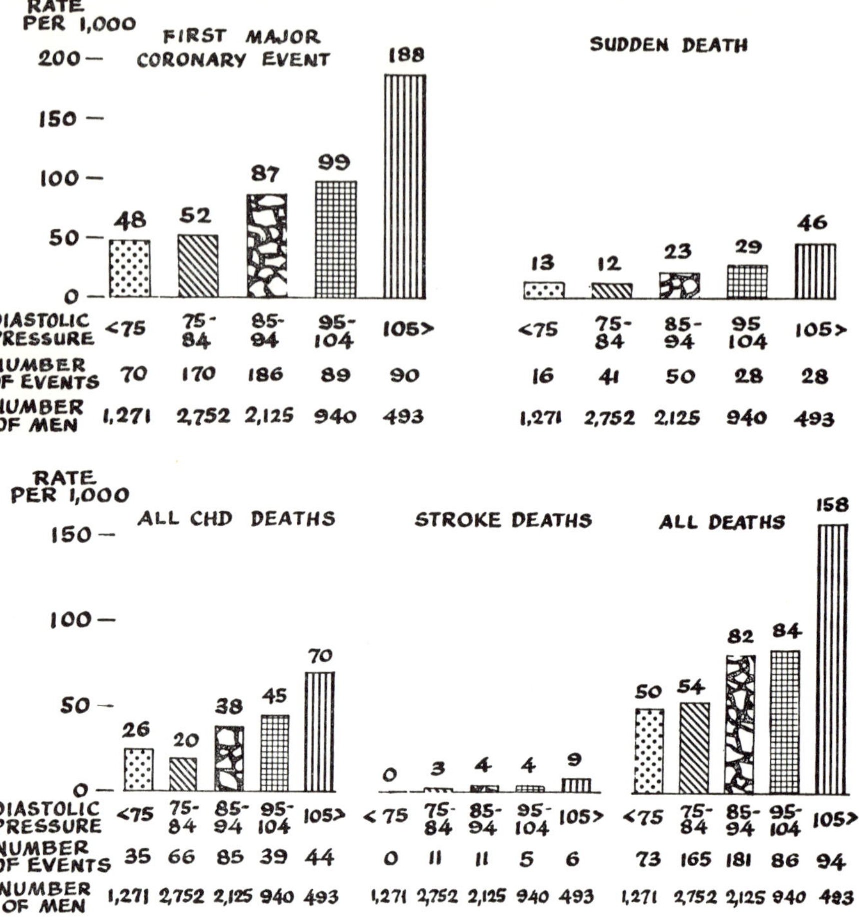

Fig. 2. National Cooperative Pooling Project; diastolic blood pressure level at entry and 10-year age-adjusted rates per 1 000 men for: first major coronary event, sudden death (upper graph), any coronary death, stroke death, death from all causes (lower graph); first major coronary event includes nonfatal MI, fatal MI, sudden death due to CHD; U.S. white males age 30–59 at entry; all rates age-adjusted by 10-year age groups to the U.S. white male population, 1960 (1, la.–m., 2).

This basic set of conclusions does not negate–but rather places in proper context–the clinical use of practical cutting points, e.g., serum cholesterol of less than 200 mg./dl. as normal; 200–249 as borderline; 250 or greater as abnormal. As American Heart Association statements on risk factors have emphasized, this 250 mg./dl. level for defining hypercholesterolemia is approximately the 2 to 1 cutting point, i.e., persons positive for this risk factor are approximately twice as susceptible to premature CHD as those with lower levels (everything else being equal). The impact of these factors is no small 10 per cent, but rather 100 per cent–a doubling of risk.

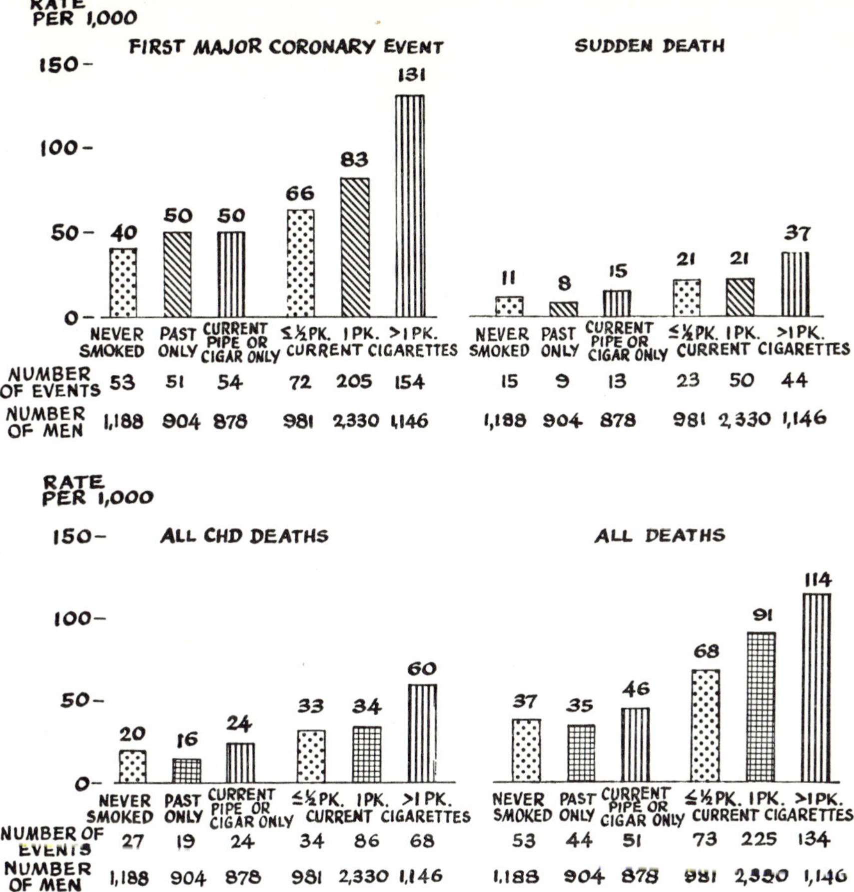

Fig. 3. National Cooperative Pooling Project; smoking status at entry and 10-year age-adjusted rates per 1 000 men for: first major coronary event, sudden death (upper graph), and coronary death, death from all causes (lower graph); first major coronary event includes nonfatal MI, fatal MI, sudden death due to CHD; U.S. white males age 30–59 at entry; all rates age-adjusted by 10-year age groups to the U.S. white male population, 1960 (1, la.–m., 2).

But as useful as this practical approach of cutting points is, it remains an oversimplification of reality. After all, a person with a serum cholesterol of 240 is at greater risk than one at 210 and he in turn is a greater risk than one at 160. How then to make use of all the quantitative information in clinical and public health practice? New methods of statistical evaluation do in fact make this possible (see below).

As for cigarette smoking, massive studies in the United States have repeatedly shown that any regular use of cigarettes is associated with increased risk of CHD (Fig. 3) (2). However, the risk for ex-cigarette smokers is about the same as for those who never smoked. The practical implications are obvious: Don't smoke cigarettes, or–if a current smoker–quit while still ahead, i.e., still free of CHD. It pays!

For those regularly smoking cigarettes when first examined, risk rose steadily with number of cigarettes smoked per day (Fig. 3). Once again, the relationship is quantitative and continuous. The gradient is twofold between those who smoke a pack or less and those smoking more than a pack. A dose-response relationship of this kind is one piece of evidence in favor of a causative relationship. Another is the consistent findings in several postmortem studies that coronary atherosclerosis was more severe in persons who had smoked cigarettes than in non-cigarette users (2). Note in Figure 3 that 60 per cent of the men are cigarette smokers. They account for no less than 431 of the 589 new events (73.2 %).

In Figure 4, the three risk factors are arranged in various combinations in order to assess their additive or synergistic predictive power (2). In this display, a single cutting point has reluctantly been used to separate "high" from "not high" levels. (N.B.: "Not high" is not equal to low or optimal–at least not for serum cholesterol and diastolic pressure, as is evident from the cutting points of 250 mg./dl. and 90 mm. Hg respectively.) As already noted, this approach is arbitrary and undesirable. However, such analyses would become impossibly complex if the variables were quantitated at several levels. As long as this limitation is kept in mind, looking at combinations of risk factors in this way is useful and informative. Newer biomathematical techniques, specifically multivariate risk functions, obviate these problems by treating risk factors as continuous, strictly quantitative variables. However, this approach has not yet been translated into clinical terms. There is a place therefore, for both kinds of display.

In Figure 4, the 7 342 Pooling Project men are divided into six of eight possible subgroups. This permits evaluation of the independent and additive effect of cigarette smoking. Thus, when the 2 018 men with cigarette smoking as the only risk factor are compared with the 1 249 men with none of the three risk factors, the 10-year rates of first major coronary events are 45 and 20 per 1 000 respectively. Cigarette smoking is associated with a more than twofold increase in risk. The situation is similar for the other two paired comparisons–cigarette smokers vs. non-cigarette smokers, with one other risk factor (1 794 and 1 302 men respectively); cigarette smokers vs. non-cigarette smokers, with two other risk factors (595 and 384 men respectively). Moreover, cigarette smoking consistently makes an independent and additive contribution to risk of sudden death, coronary death, and death from all causes.

Similar analyses also demonstrate that serum cholesterol and blood pres-

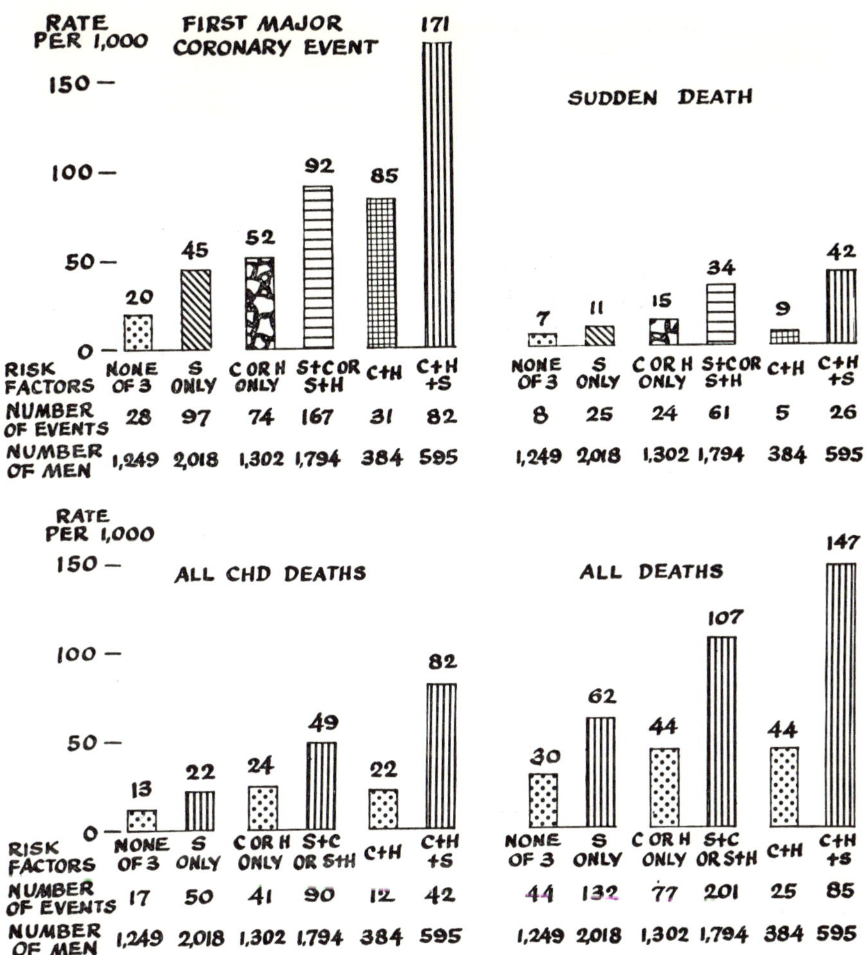

Fig. 4. National Cooperative Pooling Projects; status with respect to three major risk factors at entry and 10-year age-adjusted rates per 1 000 men for: first major coronary event, sudden death (upper graph), and coronary death, death from all causes (lower graph); first major coronary event includes nonfatal MI, fatal MI, sudden death due to CHD; U.S. white males age 30–59 at entry; all rates age-adjusted by 10-year age groups to the U.S. white male population, 1960; rates presented are for non-cigarette smokers vs. cigarette smokers at entry with simultaneous control of blood pressure and serum cholesterol level; the following cutting points were used: cigarette smoking (S), any use at entry; serum cholesterol (C), 250 mg./dl; diastolic blood pressure (H), 90 mm.Hg (1, 1a.–m., 2).
(1, 1a.–m., 2).

sure–like cigarette smoking–each make an independent and additive contribution to risk.

In Figure 5, the same data are again displayed, in simpler form, so that the three risk factors are not distinguished one from the other (2). Once again it is worth noting: the analysis is a crude one in that each man is

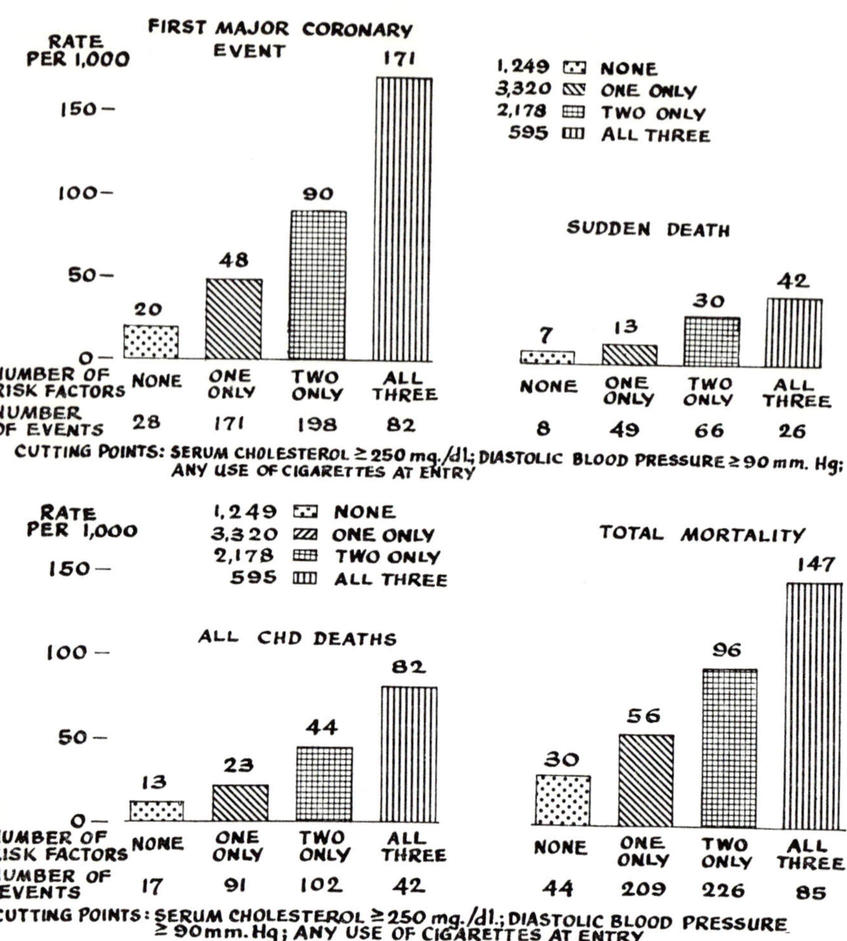

Fig. 5. National Cooperative Pooling Project; status with respect to combinations of three major risk factors at entry (serum cholesterol, diastolic blood pressure, cigarette smoking) and 10-year age-adjusted rates per 1 000 men for: first major coronary event, sudden death (upper graph) any coronary death, death from all causes (lower graph); first major coronary event includes nonfatal MI, fatal MI, sudden death due to CHD; U.S. white males, age 30–59 at entry; all rates age-adjusted by 10-year age groups to the U.S. white male population, 1960 (1, la.–m., 2).

characterized only on the basis of a single measurement of each risk factor at the entry examination, and his status with respect to each factor is arrived at by dichotomization (high or not high). Nevertheless the subgroups were very different in their 10-year morbidity and mortality experience. Presence of only one risk factor—as compared to none—was associated with a substantial increase (2.4 fold, or 140 %) in probability of a major coronary event over the next decade. Increase in risk of a fatal event, including total mortality, was almost double. For the men with any two of the risk factors, risk of a major event was increased more than fourfold; risk of death, more than threefold. For the men with all three factors, risk of a major event was increased more than eightfold; risk of death, fivefold. This is indeed powerful prediction from three simple variables, measured once, and simply dichotomized—far more powerful prediction than is available for most other diseases, acute or chronic!

Note further the typical American situation, product of our way of life: only 1 249 of the 7 342 white males age 30–59 at entry—i.e., only 17 per cent—were classified not high for all three factors. All the rest had one or more risk factors: 45 per cent with one, 30 per cent with two, 8 per cent with all three. These latter two subgroups, with any two or all three risk factors (38 % of the total group), accounted for 58 per cent of first major coronary events, 62 per cent of sudden death, 57 per cent of coronary deaths, 55 per cent of all deaths.

Obviously it is appropriate to designate persons with such combinations of these traits as very high risk individuals, very prone to premature atherosclerotic disease. Obviously too, especially since a first event is so often a catastrophic one (25 % are sudden deaths), it is very sound strategy to detect such very high risk men as early in young adulthood and middle age as possible, and to assist them preventively by bringing about sustained correction of their risk factors, by safe well-tested means—nutritional for hypercholesterolemia, hygienic for cigarette smoking, nutritional (weight control and moderate salt restriction) plus pharmacologic (when necessary) for hypertension.

Acknowledgments

It is a pleasure to acknowledge the cooperation and support of Eric Oldberg, M.D., Chairman, Board of Directors, Chicago Health Research Foundation. It is also a pleasure to express appreciation to the staff of the Chicago Health Research Foundation aiding in this research, especially the author's senior colleagues in the long-term study in the Peoples Gas Company: David M. Berkson, M.D., Howard A. Lindberg, M.D., Richard B. Shekelle, Ph.D., Rose Stamler, M.A.; also Howard Adler, Ph.D., Morton B. Epstein, Ph.D., Roberta Crawford, Nancy Dalton, Wanda Drake, Celene Epstein, Dana King, Cecelia Kohorst, W. H. McAtee, Wilda A. Miller, Frances Petersen, Margie Shores, Betty Stevens and Eka Tomashewsky. We are also grateful to P. Meier, Ph.D., of the Department of Statistics and the Biological Sciences Computation Center, University of Chicago. It is also a pleasure to express appreciation to the Peoples Gas, Light and Coke Company, its Chairman Remick McDowell, its President Ward McCallister, its officers and the staff of its Medical Department for their invaluable cooperation.

The research has been supported by the American Heart Association, Chicago Heart Association, and the National Heart and Lung Institute, National Institutes of Health, United States Public Health Service.

References

1. Data from the Pooling Project, Council on Epidemiology, American Heart Association—a national cooperative project for pooling data from the Albany civil servant, Chicago Peoples Gas Company, Chicago Western Electric Company, Framingham community. Los Angeles civil servant. Minneapolis-St. Paul business men, Tecumseh community, and U.S. railroad men prospective epidemiologic studies of adult cardiovascular disease in the United States. The following are representative references on the individual studies and on the results on the Pooling Project presented to date:

1 a. Doyle, J. T.: Risk Factors in Coronary Heart Disease. *New York State J. Med. 63*: 1317, 1963.

1 b. Stamler, J.: Cardiovascular Diseases in the United States. *Amer. J. Cardiol. 10*: 319, 1962.

1 c. Paul, O., Lepper, M. J., Phelan, W. H., Dupertuis, G. W. MacMillan, A., McKean, H. & Park, H.: A Longitudinal Study of Coronary Heart Disease. *Circulation 28*: 20, 1963.

1 d. Dawber, T. R., Kannel, W. B. & McNamara, P. M.: The Prediction of Coronary Heart Disease. *Trans. Assoc. Life Insur. Med. Dir. Amer. 47:* 70, 1964.

1 e. Chapman, J. M. & Massey, F. J.: The Interrelationship of Serum Cholesterol, Hypertension, Body Weight, and Risk of Coronary Disease. Results of the First Ten Years Follow-up in the Los Angeles Heart Study. *J. Chron. Dis. 17:* 933, 1964.

1 f. Keys, A., Taylor, H. L., Blackburn, H., Brozek, J., Anderson, J. T. & Simonson, E.: Coronary Heart Disease among Minnesota Business and Professional Men Followed Fifteen Years. *Circulation 28:* 381, 1963.

1 g. Epstein, F. H., Ostrander, L. D., Jr., Johnson, B. C., Payne, M. W. Hayner, N. S., Keller, J. B. & Francis, T., Jr.: Epidemiological Studies of Cardiovascular Disease in a Total Community—Tecumseh, Michigan. *Ann. Intern. Med. 62:* 1170, 1965.

1 h. Taylor, H. L., Blackburn, H., Keys, A., Parlin, R. W., Vasquez, C. & Puchner, T.: IV. Five-Year Follow-up of Employees of Selected U.S. Railroad Companies (ed. A. Keys). Coronary Heart Disease in Seven Countries. *Circulation 41*: Suppl. I–20, 1970.

1 i. Moore, F. E.: Some Preliminary Findings from the Pooling Project of the Council on Epidemiology, American Heart Association. Paper Presented at the Conference on Cardiovascular Disease Epidemiology, Council on Epidemiology, American Heart Association, March 3–4, 1969, New Orleans, La.

1 j. Doyle, J. T. & Kinch, S. H.: Coronary Heart Disease in the United States: Some Preliminary Findings from the Pooling Project of the Council on Epidemiology of the American Heart Association. Presented at the 42nd Scientific Sessions, American Heart Association, Nov. 14, 1969.

1 k. Epstein, F. H. & Moore, F. E.: Progress Report to the National Heart Institute on the National Cooperative Pooling Project, 1968.

1 l. Paul, O.: Risks of mild hypertension: A ten-year report. *Brit. Heart J. 33:* Suppl., 116, 1971.

1 m. Doyle, J. T. & Kannel, W. B.: Coronary Risk Factors: 10 Year Findings in 7, 446 Americans. Pooling Project, Council on Epidemiology, American Heart Association. Paper presented to the VI World Congress of Cardiology, London, England, Sept. 1970.

2. Inter-Society Commission for Heart Disease Resources. Atherosclerosis Study Group and Epidemiology Study Group. Primary Prevention of the Atherosclerotic Diseases. *Circulation 42:* A55, 1970.

The natural history of myocardial infarction in the Coronary Drug Project. Prognostic indicators following infarction

The Coronary Drug Project Research Group

By Henry Blackburn, Paul Canner, William Krol, Suketami Tominaga and Jeremiah Stamler

Factors related to mortality following myocardial infarction (MI) have been studied in the Coronary Drug Project (CDP), a Collaborative Study of the United States National Heart and Lung Institute. This is a large-scale double-blind clinical trial of the effectiveness and safety of lipid lowering drugs compared to a placebo in reducing mortality or reinfarction (1). The men were survivors (at least 3 months; average 3 years) of one or more documented MI and were ages 30–64 at entry. All had a fair to good functional recovery (New York Heart Association Class I or II), were free of a specified list of life-threatening diseases, and were neither on anti-coagulant therapy, nor, if diabetic, on insulin.

The "natural history" of coronary heart disease (CHD) in these MI survivors is under detailed investigation among the 2 788 cases randomly assigned to the placebo group. This report considers the relationship of entry characteristics of the placebo-treated men to their subsequent mortality experience during the following-up period of 1 to 5 years (average 18 months for baseline clinical characteristics, 30 months for ECG findings). Death was ascribed to CHD in over 75 % of cases and was sudden in over 40 %.

The structure of the CDP is indicated in the extensive list of acknowledgements. This organizational framework is considered necessary in the United States for optimal operation and quality control of a clinical trial. Details of the CDP design and method, along with more complete results are given in other publications (1, 2, 3, 4).

Several types of analysis were made to relate the baseline or entry characteristics to the subsequent mortality experience during the follow-up period. In Figure 1 along the abscissa is the baseline measure or risk factor, in this case increasing age at entry of the MI patient. The number of men with each class of risk variable at entry is given as a denominator, and the proportion of total deaths during the follow-up period are plotted in the vertical bars. The lines is the best fit of a straight line to the data using a linear regression in which the dependent variable, y, is mortality (0 or 1) and the independent variable, x, is the actual age at baseline. The t_l value is the slope (the regression coefficient) divided by its standard error, ignoring all other factors besides the variable x (age). The t_s value does the same for the contribution of x (age) when the regression is solved for the following multiple variables simultaneously:

Age
Systolic blood pressure
Diastolic blood pressure
One-hour glucose tolerance
Serum cholesterol
Serum triglycerides
Relative body weight
Serum uric acid
Cigarette smoking habit
New York Heart Association functional class
CDP risk class (acute phase severity)
Number of prior MI
Interval since last MI
Heart size on chest *X*ray
Congestive failure history
Digitalis therapy history
Angina pectoris history
Intermittent claudication history
ECG findings by Minnesota Code.

Similar analysis has been made for specific cohorts of cases, including all men with completed follow-up for 1, 2, or 3 years. Results are quite comparable to those for total mortality in the study to date. Life table analyses which utilize the experience of all men, according to their duration of survival in the placebo group, show similar results. Other multivariate models than the least squares solution, including the Truett-Cornfield (5) and Walker-Duncan models (6), have been used with these data, and the distribution of risk scores for the survivors and the dead are generally very similar to those in the linear model. Simple two-way analysis is reported elsewhere in detail, in which the prognostic importance of each of these baseline characteristics was examined within groups high and low with respect to one other variable at a time (3, 4).

Results

Figure 1 shows that mortality during an average 18 months follow-up was importantly related to age, being 60 % higher in the older than in the younger group. However, the adjusted t value suggests that this clear crude

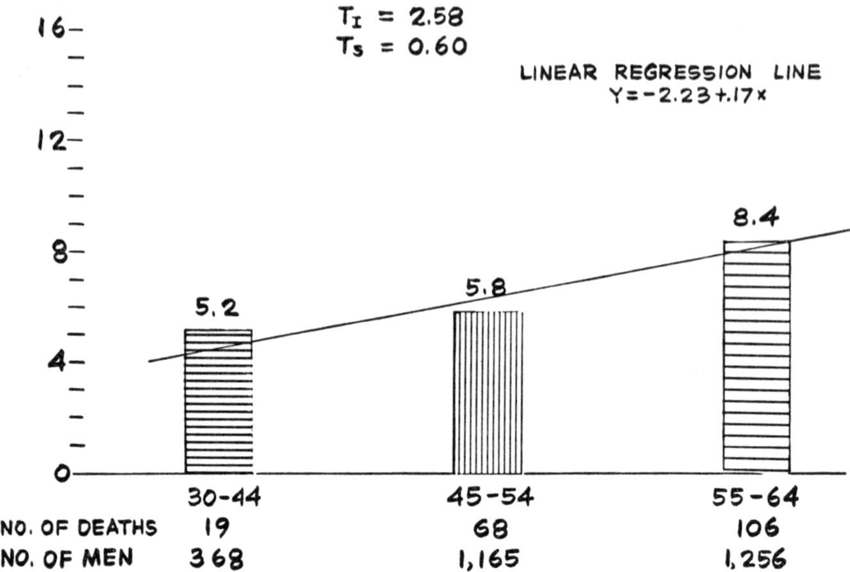

Fig. 1. Relationship between age at entry and mortality, placebo group, Coronary Drug Project; average duration of follow-up is 18 months; T_I is the simple or unadjusted t value, T_S is the t value adjusted for 15 other baseline variables.

relationship is apparently due to factors associated with age rather than to age itself.

This analysis was carried out for all individual and combined risk characteristics and revealed crude prognostic importance, with a significant excess mortality, for the following clinical characteristics of MI patients:

Cardiac enlargement
New York Heart Association functional class II
Three or more prior MI
History of heart failure or digitalis-diuretic therapy
History of angina pectoris
History of intermittent claudication.

Figure 2 shows that using simple clinical classifications of MI survivors, it is possible to discriminate between patients with a 9-fold difference in risk of mortality, i.e. between patients with less than 2 % mortality risk versus over 16 % risk (in 18 months).

Of the 8 clinical characteristics, all but functional class appear to be independently predictive when associated variables are considered simultaneously.

Crude predictive importance was found for the following measured baseline variables in the CDP men:

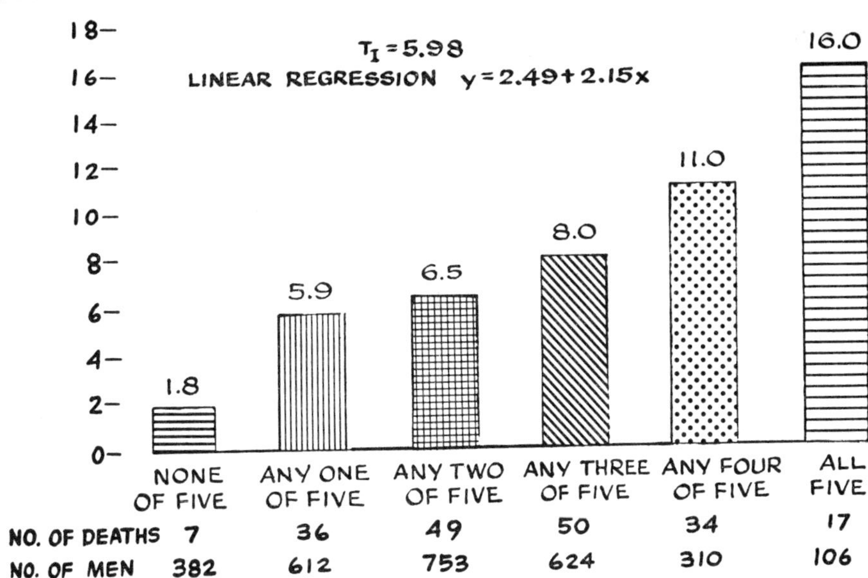

Fig. 2. Age, risk, angina, New York Heart Association class, history of congestive heart failure at entry and mortality, placebo group, Coronary Drug Project; average duration of follow-up is 18 months; T_I is the unadjusted t value.

Age
Systolic blood pressure and pulse pressure level
1-hour glucose tolerance value
Serum cholesterol value
Degree of ECG ST segment depression.

The contribution of age was no longer significant after adjustment was made for variables associated with age. The others appeared to retain their independent prognostic importance, and the greatest mortality difference was associated with ST segment depression in the baseline resting ECG.

The following items had so far in this early follow-up experience, no important prognostic power:
Relative body weight
Diastolic blood pressure level
Serum triglyceride level
Cigarette smoking intensity.

Figure 3 a is an attempt to dissect the relative importance and possible interaction of serum cholesterol and triglyceride levels in prognosis following infarction. The arbitrary values depicted for increasing cholesterol level, within low, moderate and high classes of triglyceride level, are multiplied by the actual regression coefficients obtained in solving the multiple

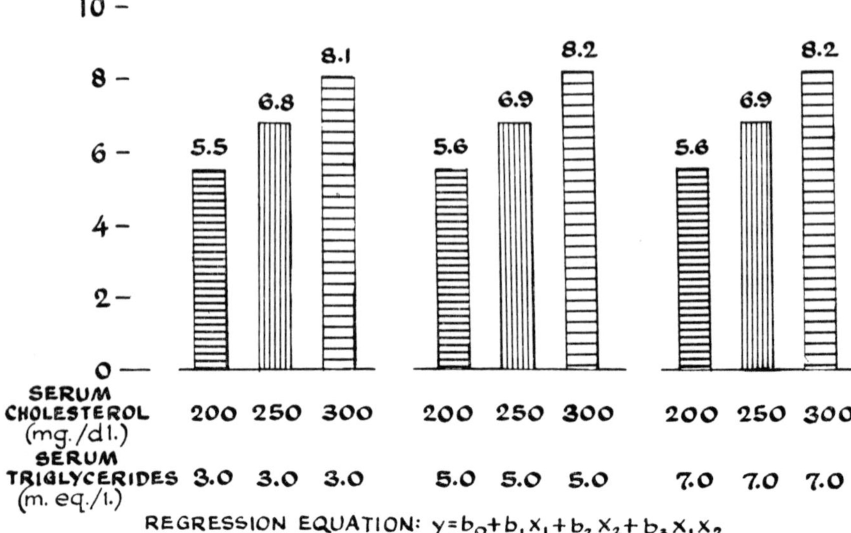

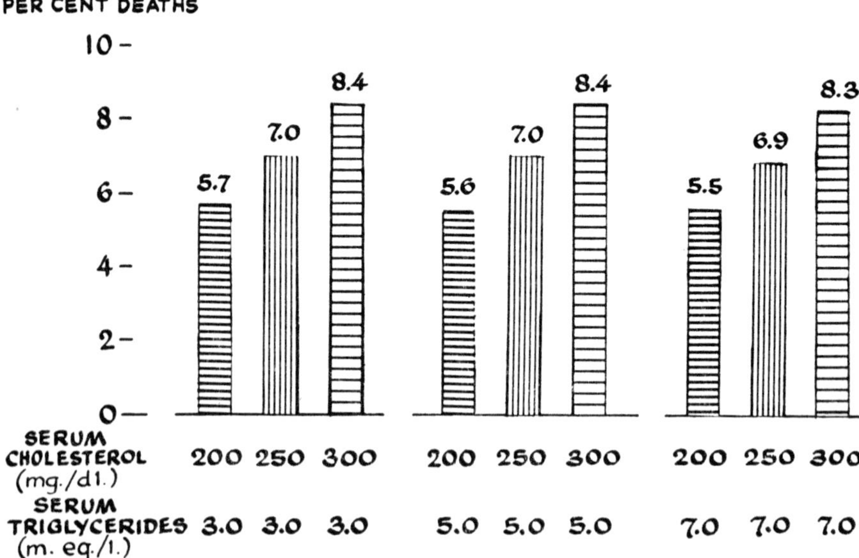

Fig. 3 a–b. Serum cholesterol, triglycerides at entry and mortality estimated from multiple regression analysis, placebo group, Coronary Drug Project; average duration of follow-up is 18 months; Figure 3 a presents points read off the multiple linear regression curve estimated without consideration of other variables; Figure 3 b presents points read off the multiple linear regression curve estimated with adjustment for other baseline factors.

linear regression for mortality in the entire CDP placebo group. This smoothed picture suggests, but does not establish, that mortality following infarction increases with serum cholesterol level for each class of triglyceride level, that mortality is unrelated to triglyceride level, and that there is no interaction between the two. A more complete analysis of these relationships is presented elsewhere (4), but Figure 3 b examines the same relationships while adjusting simultaneously for the other clinical characteristics.

Discussion

A single standardized assessment of baseline clinical characteristics among selected MI survivors with good functional recovery disclosed a number which are significantly related to subsequent risk of dying. Several types of analysis indicated that clinical and ECG evidence of myocardial ischemia, conduction defect, cardiac enlargement, and a history of heart failure or intermittent claudication are very important indicators of prognosis. Serum cholesterol and blood pressure are statistically significant risk indicators but are apparently much weaker prognostically after, compared to before, the first MI. Relative weight and cigarette smoking were, so far, insignificant risk indicators.

The natural history experience in the CDP is still early, and the results must be considered tentative. Moreover, interpretation of the multivariate analyses is not yet certain. However, there appears to be evidence here that 1) infarct survivors can be identified having vastly different risk of mortality in a given period 2) and that the usual "primary risk factors" are much less important after MI than before. The public health implication is clear; the greater advantage is to be expected the earlier an attempt is made to modify risk factors.

References

1. Coronary Drug Project Research Group, Report of the. The Coronary Drug Project. Initial findings leading to modifications of its research protocol. *J.A.M.A. 214*: 1303–1313, 1970.
2. Coronary Drug Project Research Group. Control of hyperlipidemia: IV. Progress in drug trials of secondary prevention, with particular reference to the Coronary Drug Project. In *Atherosclerosis: Second International Symposium* (ed. R. J. Jones), p. 382. Springer-Verlag, New York, 1970.
3. Coronary Drug Project Research Group, Report of the. Prepared by H. Blackburn and S. Tominaga. *The natural history of myocardial infarction. The prognostic importance of the electrocardiogram following infarction,* Annals of Internal Medicine. In press.

4. Coronary Drug Project Research Group, Report of the. Prepared by J. Stamler, W. Krol and P. Canner. The natural history of myocardial infarction. *The prognostic importance of serum lipids following infarction.* In press.
5. Truett, J., Cornfield, J. & Kannel, W.: A multivariate analysis of the risk of coronary heart disease in Framingham. *J. Chron. Dis. 20:* 511, 1967.
6. Walker, S. H. & Duncan, D. B.: Estimation of the probability of an event as a function of several independent variables. *Biometrika 54:* 167, 1967.

Acknowledgements

The effective execution of the Coronary Drug Project depends on the efforts of the following key bodies and their senior staff:

Policy Board
Robert W. Wilkins, M.D. (Chairman), University Hospital Boston
Jacob E. Bearman, Ph.D., University of Minnesota, Minneapolis
Edwin Boyle, M.D., Miami Heart Institute, Miami Beach
Louis Lasagna, M.D., University of Rochester, Rochester, New York
William M. Smith, M.D., USPHS, San Francisco
Christian R. Klimt, M.D., Dr P.H. (ex officio), University of Maryland, Baltimore
Jeremiah Stamler, M.D. (ex officio), Chicago Health Research Foundation, Chicago

Steering Committee
Jeremiah Stamler, M.D. (Chairman), Chicago Health Research Foundation, Chicago
Kenneth Berge, M.D., Mayo Clinic, Rochester, Minnesota
William Bernstein, M.D., Mount Sinai Hospital, Miami Beach
Henry Blackburn, M.D., University of Minnesota, Minneapolis
Gerald R. Cooper, M.D., Center for Disease Control, Atlanta
Jerome Cornfield, University of Pittsburgh, Bethesda, Maryland
Nicholas J. Galluzzi, M.D., USPHS Hospital, Staten Island, New York
Max Halperin, Ph.D., NHLI, Bethesda, Maryland
Christian R. Klimt, M.D., Dr P.H., University of Maryland, Baltimore
Charles A. Laubach, Jr., M.D., Geisinger Medical Foundation, Danville, Pa.
Bernard I. Lewis, M.D., Palo Alto Medical Research Foundation, Palo Alto, Calif.
Jessie Marmorston, M.D., University of Southern California, Los Angeles
William B. Parsons, Jr., M.D., Jackson Clinic, Madison, Wisconsin
Milton Nichaman, M.D., USPHS Hospital, San Francisco, California (1967–1969)
Henry K. Schoch, M.D., VA Hospital, Ann Arbor, Michigan (1967–1969)

Coordinating Center (University of Maryland, Baltimore, Maryland)
Christian R. Klimt, M.D., Director
Curtis Meinert, Ph.D., Deputy Director
Paul Canner, Ph.D., Chief Statistician
Elizabeth Heinz, Research Analyst
Genell Knatterud, Ph.D., Statistician
William Krol, Ph.D., Statistician
Suketami Tominaga, M.D., Epidemiologist-cardiologist

Central Laboratory (USPHS Communicable Disease Center, Atlanta, Georgia)
Gerald Cooper, M.D., Medical Director
Adrian Hainline, Jr., M.D., Chief
Eloise Eavenson, Ph.D.
Alan Mather, Ph.D.
Mrs Sara Gill

ECG Center (University of Minnesota, Minneapolis)
Henry Blackburn, M.D., Director
Robin MacGregor, Chief Technician

National Heart and Lung Institute Staff (Bethesda, Maryland)
Theodore Cooper, M.D., Director
Robert Ringler, M.D., Deputy Director
William Zukel, M.D., Associate Director, Clinical Applications
Max Halperin, Ph.D., Statistician
William Friedewald, M.D., Statistician
Eleanore Darby, Ph.D., Administrator
Michael Davidson, M.D., Liaison Officer
William Vicic, M.D., Assistant Liaison Officer

Public Health Service, Supply Service Center
Salvatore Gasdia, Officer in Charge

Data and Safety Monitoring Committee
Curtis Meinert, Ph.D. (Co-Chairman), University of Maryland, Baltimore
Jeremiah Stamler, M.D. (Co-Chairman), Chicago Health Research Foundation, Chicago
E. Cowles Andrus, M.D., Johns Hopkins University, Baltimore
Henry Blackburn, M.D., University of Minnesota, Minneapolis
Paul L. Canner, Ph.D., University of Maryland, Baltimore
Thomas Chalmers, M.D., NHLI, Bethesda, Maryland
Jerome Cornfield, University of Pittsburgh, Bethesda, Maryland
James R. Gillette, Ph.D., NHLI, Bethesda, Maryland
Adrian Hainline, Ph.D., Center for Disease Control, Atlanta
Max Halperin, Ph.D., NHLI, Bethesda, Maryland
Gerald Klatskin, M.D., Yale University, New Haven, Connecticut
Christian R. Klimt, M.D., Dr P.H., University of Maryland, Baltimore
Robert I. Levy, M.D., NHLI, Bethesda, Maryland
Elliot Newman, M.D., Vanderbilt University, Nashville, Tennessee
Medical Liaison Officer*, NHLI, Bethesda, Maryland

---

* The following persons have served as Medical Liaison Officer during the course of the CDP:

John Turner, M.D. (1962–1963)
Starr Ford, M.D. (1963–1965)
Clifford Bachrach, M.D. (1965–1966)
Terrence Fisher, M.D. (1966–1967)
Hubert Loncin, M.D. (1967–1968)
Howard Marsh, M.D. (1968–1969)
Richard Havlik, M.D. (1969–1970)
Thomas Landau, M.D. (1970–1971)
Michael Davidson, M.D. (1971–1972)
William Vicic, M.D. (1972–1973)

Fred Ederer, NHLI, Bethesda, Maryland (1968–1970)
William Friedewald, M.D., NHLI, Bethesda, Maryland

Criterion Subcommittee
Nicholas J. Galluzzi, M.D. (Chairman), USPHS Hospital, Staten Island, New York
Kenneth Berge, M.D., Mayo Clinic, Rochester, Minnesota
Henry Blackburn, M.D., University of Minnesota, Minneapolis
Medical Liaison Officer*, NHLI, Bethesda, Maryland

Laboratory Subcommittee
Adrian Hainline, Ph.D. (Co-Chairman), Center for Disease Control, Atlanta
Christian R. Klimt, M.D., Dr P.H., (Co-Chairman), University of Maryland, Baltimore
Paul L. Canner, Ph.D., University of Maryland, Baltimore
Gerald R. Cooper, M.D., Center for Disease Control, Atlanta
William Krol, Ph.D., University of Maryland, Baltimore
Alan Mather, Ph.D., Center of Disease Control, Atlanta
Curtis L. Meinert, Ph.D., University of Maryland, Baltimore
Jeremiah Stamler, M.D., Chicago Health Research Foundation, Chicago
Medical Liaison Officer*, NHLI, Bethesda, Maryland

Editorial Review Board
Jeremiah Stamler, M.D. (Chairman), Chicago Healt Research Foundation, Chicago
Kenneth Berge, M.D., Mayo Clinic, Rochester, Minnesota
Henry Blackburn, M.D., University of Minnesota, Minneapolis
Jerome Cornfield, University of Pittsburgh, Bethesda, Maryland
Christian R. Klimt, M.D., Dr P.H., University of Maryland, Baltimore
Robert W. Wilkins, M.D., University Hospitals, Boston
Medical Liaison Officer*, NHLI, Bethesda, Maryland

Statistical Subcommittee
Paul L. Canner, Ph.D. (Co-Chairman), University of Maryland, Baltimore
Max Halperin, Ph.D. (Co-Chairman), NHLI, Bethesda, Maryland
Jerome Cornfield, University of Pittsburgh, Bethesda, Maryland
William Friedewald, M.D., NHLI, Bethesda, Maryland
Christian R. Klimt, M.D., Dr P.H. University of Maryland, Baltimore
Genell Knatterud, Ph.D., University of Maryland, Baltimore
William Krol, Ph.D., University of Maryland, Baltimore
Curtis L. Meinert, Ph.D., University of Maryland, Baltimore

Natural History Study Committee
Henry Blackburn, M.D. (Co-Chairman), University of Minnesota, Minneapolis
Jeremiah Stamler, M.D. (Co-Chairman), Chicago Health Research Foundation, Chicago
Kenneth G. Berge, M.D., Mayo Clinic, Rochester, Minnesota
David M. Berkson, M.D., St. Joseph Hospital, Chicago
William H. Bernstein, M.D., Mount Sinai Hospital, Miami Beach
Paul L. Canner, Ph.D., University of Maryland, Baltimore
Jerome Cornfield, University of Pittsburgh, Bethesda, Maryland

Irving, Ershler, M.D., University of Utah, Salt Lake City
Charles K. Friedberg, M.D., Mount Sinai Hospital, New York
William Friedewald, M.D., NHLI, Bethesda, Maryland
Max Halperin, Ph.D., NHLI, Bethesda, Maryland
Christian R. Klimt, M.D., Dr P.H., University of Maryland, Baltimore
William Krol, Ph.D., University of Maryland, Baltimore
Curtis, Meinert, Ph.D., University of Maryland, Baltimore
Bernard Tabatznik, M.D., Sinai Hospital, Baltimore
Suketami Tominaga, M.D., University of Maryland, Baltimore
William J. Zukel, M.D., NHLI, Bethesda, Maryland
Medical Liaison Officer*, NHLI, Bethesda, Maryland

Principal Investigators, Clinic Research Centers
Kenneth G. Berge, M.D., Mayo Clinic, Rochester, Minnesota (1)
Nicholas Galluzzi, M.D., USPHS Hospital, Staten Island, New York (2)
Jessie Marmorston, M.D., University of Southern California, Los Angeles (3)
James A. Schoenberger, M.D., Presbyterian St. Luke's Hospital, Chicago (4)
Samuel Baer, M.D., Albert Einstein Medical Center, Philadelphia (5)
Henry K. Schoch, M.D., Ann Arbor Hospital Group, Ann Arbor, Michigan (6)
J. Richard Warbasse, M.D., USPHS Hospital, Baltimore (7)
Robert M. Kohn, M.D., Buffalo General Hospital, Buffalo, New York (8)
Bernard I. Lewis, M.D., Palo Alto Medical Clinic and Research Foundation, Palo Alto (9)
Richard J. Jones, M.D., University of Chicago, Chicago (10)
Kenneth Hyatt, M.D., USPHS Hospital, San Francisco (11)
Dean A. Emanuel, M.D., Marshfield Clinic, Marshfield, Wisconsin (12)
David Z. Morgan, M.D., West Virginia University, Morgantown (13)
Jeremiah Stamler, M.D., St. Joseph Hospital, Chicago (14)
William H. Bernstein, M.D., Mount Sinai Hospital, Miami Beach, Florida (15)
Ernst Greif, M.D., Maimonides Medical Center, Brooklyn, New York (16)
James K. Conrad, M.D., Lovelace Foundation, Albuquerque (17)
Charles K. Friedberg, M.D., Mount Sinai Hospital, New York (18)
Jacob I. Haft, M.D., Veterans Administration Hospital, Bronx, New York (19)
Gordon L. Maurice, M.D., Providence Hospital, Portland, Oregon (20)
Robert J. Myerberg, M.D., Veterans Administration Hospital, Miami (21)
Irving M. Liebow, M.D., Case Western Reserve University, Cleveland (22)
Reuben Berman, M.D., Mount Sinai Hospital, Minneapolis (23)
Charles B. Moore, M.D., Ochsner Clinic, New Orleans (24)
William B. Parsons, Jr., M.D., Jackson Clinic and Foundation, Madison, Wisc. (25)
Olga M. Haring, M.D., Northwestern University, Chicago (26)
Robert C. Schlant, M.D., Emory University School of Medicine, Grady Memorial Hospital, Atlanta, Georgia (27)
Joseph A. Wagner, M.D., Bryn Mawr Hospital, Bryn Mawr, Pennsylvania (29)
Ward Laramore, M.D., Veterans Administration Hospital, Indianapolis (30)
Donald McCaughan, M.D., Veterans Administration Hospital, West Roxbury, Massachusetts (31)
Robert W. Oblath, M.D., St. Joseph Hospital Medical Center, Burbank, Calif. (32)

Peter C. Gazes, M.D., Medical University of South Carolina, Charleston (33)
Bernard Tabatznik, M.D., Sinai Hospital of Baltimore, Baltimore (34)
Leo Elson, M.D., University and V. A. Hospitals, Jackson, Mississippi (35)
Mario Garcia-Palmieri, M.D., University of Puerto Rico, San Juan (36)
Donald Berkowitz, M.D., Sidney Hillman Medical Center, Philadelphia (37)
Robert L. Grissom, M.D., University of Nebraska, Omaha (38)
Ralph C. Scott, University of Cincinnati Medical Center, Cincinnati (39)
Arthur J. Gosselin, M.D., Miami Heart Institute, Miami Beach (40)
Charles A. Laubach, Jr., M.D., Geisinger Medical Foundation, Danville, Pennsylvania (41)
Ralph E. Cole. M.D., Medical Associates Research Foundation, Chelmsford, Massachusetts (42)
Thaddeus E. Prout, M.D., Greater Baltimore Medical Center, Baltimore (43)
Bernard A. Sachs, M.D., Montefiore Hospital and Medical Center, Bronx (44)
Donald L. Warkentin, M.D., University of Iowa Hospital, Iowa City (45)
C. Basil Williams, M.D., Ogden Research Foundation, Ogden, Utah (46)
Stephen J. Herbert, M.D., USPHS Hospital, New Orleans (47)
Fred I. Gilbert, Jr., M.D., Straub Medical Research Institute, Honolulu (48)
Sidney A. Levine, M.D., Melrose-Wakefield Hospital, Melrose, Mass. (50)
Louis B. Matthew, Jr., M.D., Hitchcock Clinic, Hanover, New Hampshire (51)
Irving Ershler, M.D., University of Utah, Salt Lake City (52)
Elmer E. Cooper, M.D., Santa Rosa Medical Center, San Antonio, Texas (53)
Allan H. Barker, M.D., Salt Lake Clinic Research Foundation, Salt Lake City (54)
Paul Samuel, M.D., Long Island Jewish Hospital, Jamaica, New York (55)

Acknowledgement is also made to the University of Minnesota students who classify the electrocardiograms of the Coronary Drug Project:

Maureen M. Ahern
Candy Amlie
Philip Broberg
Karen Brugger
Andy Carley
Bill Carlson
Fred Carlson
Mary Chrun
Jane Ann Cochlin
Randall D. Cone
Susan Dorothy Dahl
Gael Davis
Tweed Ann Finlayson
Gretchen Flach
Linda Hoffman
Elizabeth Ann Kubiak
Kathleen Kupcho
Robin MacGregor
Judi Matheson
Jan Nelson
Lois Pogin
Doug Thorsen

The helpful collaboration is acknowledged of Prof. Olivier Jeanneret, Institute of Social and Preventive Medicine, University of Geneva, Switzerland, where some of this material was written up, under the excellent Sabattical leave facilities provided.

This collaborative study is fully supported by research grants and other funds from the National Heart and Lung Institute.

Discussion

Risk factors—cause or effect?

Lars Werkö (Chairman) opened the discussion by asking Jerry Morris what came into his mind when he heard that there was a 50 per cent higher incidence of myocardial infarction in the men studied in the United States than in the cohorts of men in Europe.

Jerry Morris said he knew that Prof. Remington, who was not on the panel, is very much interested in the predictive capacity of the multiple logistic equation and other discriminant functions and in the reason it works less well when applied to other data. This recalled to his mind discussions over the years in his own research with his own statistical colleges. They came to the conclusion that the reason for using this method in order to bring together the variables of interest is that no better method has been discovered. The fact is that this has little to do with our picture as to how coronary heart disease develops. The multiple logistic equation doesn't really allow for acute factors versus chronic factors or for the interaction of various factors. And this is not the way he saw the build-up of coronary atherosclerosis and ischaemic heart disease. He wondered whether in fact the disappointment he had in prediction may not be due to the fact that we still lack a very good mathematical model.

Lars Werkö asked if Prof. Keys would like to comment.

Ancel Keys showed a slide and said the point he would like to make here is that such devices as the multiple logistic equation or other multivariant methods are not designed to show etiology and prove the mechanism behind the development of the disease. These devices can be used to find the people who are most at risk so that possibly something can be done about their excessive risk. Also it is useful in this way to find people who are least at risk so that their fears may be allayed. He explained that both the multiple logistic and the multiple regression equations are discriminant functions but are quite different in their mathematical characteristics. However, in practice he found that the two approaches end up with substantially the same answers. He had found no cases where it could be shown that one equation is superior to the other in discriminating or predicting the incidence of coronary heart disease. He was pleased that with only four variables it proved possible to differentiate groups of individuals which differed as much as 30–40 times in the incidence rate of the disease within the succeeding five years.

Lars Werkö asked whether the real question bothering Jerry Morris was that the multivariate analysis is a purely statistical way of looking at the problem, an approach which involves no idea about what is happening to the people concerned or what may be the clinical history of myocardial infarction. The situation is that we start with measuring four variables and we now know that within a couple of years certain persons have a 20 per cent chance of dying. But does that help you in your clinical treatment of the patients?

Jerry Stamler said that a key question in regard to the use of this approach is whether the set of coefficients generated in one study which so beautifully classify men in that study usefully predict in another study? Jerry Morris used the word "disappointment" but Dr Stamler thought that is incorrect. When, for example, the set of coefficients from the Framingham study, published in the Journal of Chronic Diseases several years ago, was applied to the Chicago Gas Company 10-years' experience, the upper quintile so classified was five times higher in the incidence rate of disease than the rate in the lowest quintile. A simple cross classification of several variables gives a similar spread in the incidence rate; it can identify groups that will differ five-fold in future incidence but those widely differing groups make up only a very small precentage of the population. The coefficients from a multiple logistic solution prove to be much more powerful than multiple cross classifications in regard to classifying men in terms of risk of future disease. So this is a powerful tool to identify high-risk subjects who then, hopefully, can be helped by efforts to control risk factors.

Lars Werkö said that Ancel Keys' data show a difference in the incidence rate of myocardial infarction in American men as compared to Europeans. If this is true it is very important. It can be a starting point for new studies. Jerry Morris was asked what he thought.

Jerry Morris said that there are a lot of other data suggesting that the incidence of coronary heart disease in the USA is greater than in Europe.

Ancel Keys said that he started his population comparisons 20 years ago with the suspicion that there were differences between populations in the incidence of this disease. This is now proved. The new major finding here is that the characteristics so far identified as risk factors do not explain more than a part of the difference in incidence of the disease. That seemed to be important in his view.

Geoffrey Rose said that he found the relatively minor defects of the prediction equation as solved in the USA to be of positive interest and not disappointing. It seemed that the logistic function applied to his own population studies serves extremely efficiently to rank the individuals in order of risk. What went wrong in the application of the European solution to the USA?. At any level of predicted risk too many cases were observed and the excess unexplained by the equation was more or less constant right across the whole range of risk. This is perhaps a clue to etiology and it might be helpful ultimately in prevention. The Americans with their unfortunate excess incidence rate suggest the need to search for some other factor, factor *X*, which is very uniform for all the American subjects in the study. It may, for example, be related to water hardness, where all the individuals in the community are approximately equally exposed; this would have quite different relevance to prevention if it did prove to be controllable. It could be that it would be easier to control such a factor *X* than personal habits.

Lars Werkö asked whether there is not also a real possibility that part of that factor *X* might be physical inactivity, because this is a characteristic which is also fairly general for the common American male.

Ancel Keys said that the multiple logistic equation had been solved including physical activity in occupation as a variable but that variable proved to have no statistical significance either in Europe or the United States. He also commented on factor *X*—something which Dr Rose suggested as being relatively uniformly spread throughout the population. That is not necessarily the case however; all that can be said here is that factor *X* cannot be very closely correlated with any of the other variables in these studies considered in the multiple logistic equation so far.

Lars A. Carlson wished consideration in this connection of triglycerides as factor *X*. From his experience with friends in the lipid field in the USA he had the impression that some types of hyperlipoprotenemia exceedingly common in the States might be related to overnutrition as well as to a low level of physical activity.

Jerry Stamler said he agreed with Dr Carlson to some extent and would say a word of caution about excluding physical activity based solely in the data about physical activity in occupation. There is much experience in the United States indicating that men classified as somewhat more active because they are in "blue collar" jobs really are no more fit in the sense of cardiopulmonary fitness than those classified as being "white collar" workers. Partly this is because the degree of additional activity in blue collar jobs in the United States is relatively small and partly because of the overwhelming effect of cigarette smoking and over-nutrition. The one prospective study so far reported in the whole world where there are measurements relevant to this question beyond physical activity at work is in Framingham where there are data on vital capacity, on heart rate, on relative weight and skinfold thickness, and an interview concerning activity outside the job. In Framingham these measures of "fitness" seemed to be related to later incidence of coronary heart disease independently of serum cholesterol, blood pressure and smoking. That set of data led Dr Stamler to have an open mind to the possibility that a more refined index of physical activity could be related to cardiopulmonary fitness and could be very important as a variable related to risk of coronary heart disease.

Jerry Stamler asked Dr Carlson if he was not struck by the fact that the Stockholm data,* as Dr Carlson showed them, give a very different picture in regard to the independent contribution of triglycerides than the data from the United States, from the original "Cooperative Study", from Dr John Gofman's later study on the west coast of the United States, and from the latest Framingham data, all of which indicate that the Sf-20-400 class of very low density lipoproteins adds nothing of predictive value over the serum cholesterol concentration. Dr Stamler also asked whether it is possible in the Stockholm study to separate and remove confounding factors due to the association between hypertriglyceridemia and hypertension.

Lars Werkö asked Prof. Remington if he would comment on the statistical questions raised by consideration of the multiple logistic results presented by Prof. Keys.

Richard Remington said he had been talking to some of Prof. Key's colleagues during the week and asking the question the answer to which was flashed on the screen today, namely how well the solution of the logistic equation from data in one study would predict in other studies. His reaction as a statistician was that the predictability was remarkably much greater and better than he would have anticipated. A difference between the total number of cases predicted and those observed is inevitable and would be expected because the coefficients in such a system of data are calculated to predict relative risk within that set of observations, not

* Not available for publication in this book

absolute risk levels as such. So it seemed to him that perhaps an underlying fact is that we may be looking at an over-all relationship that is up in the United States and down in Europe and yet the over-all regression surface, if you would put it that way, is fairly well intact in these data. If the relative predictability is compared, there is a difference in level which in a sense is itself probably quite predictable. But the encouraging thing for Prof. Remington was that within a number of different populations a single set of coefficients apparently can be used to identify the group of men with highest risk within the population. Of course Prof. Keys' quite proper cautions shoulb be noted; it is still only possible to predict 50 per cent of the cases. The fact of the matter is that those cases are being located along the multivariate surface rather well.

Another comment could be made in respect to Prof. Morris's remark about curvature and interaction between risk factors. We could, if we wish, add cross-product terms, second degree terms and things of that sort. Such items could be built into the solution. There was, in fact, some evidence of a little curvature in the USA data when applied to some of the other populations by Prof. Keys. Professor Remington would be a little reluctant to add such items because in his experience such cross-product terms and such higher degree terms confuse as much as they add to out understanding.

Lars Werkö thanked Prof. Remington and noted that Dr Gösta Tibblin had another risk factor to mention.

Gösta Tibblin said that psychosocial factors should be considered as one of the *X*-factors. They had not been studied in the investigations mentioned in this Symposium but there are investigations which show that psychosocial factors can be independent of other risk factors.

Lars Werkö remarked that it is very easy to say that we should include psychosocial factors but they are very difficult to study and almost impossible to quantitate.

Gösta Tibblin thought it is possible to quantitate these variables. He thought that we can now ask questions about "life changes". Also behaviour patterns A and B can be identified.

Lars Werkö noted that Ancel Keys had been around looking at people on Crete and Corfu and in East Finland and he asked about the situation in different countries. Are there differences in psychosocial circumstances?

Ancel Keys replied that there are indeed differences. The population groups chosen for study show contrasts in some respects in their life style, but he had no idea how to measure such differences. He thought many years ago that something could be done about measurement but he was no less sanguine about it. He would like to invite Gösta Tibblin to go to these different places and give some hints about what to do in regard to measurements of psychosocial factors and life changes.

Lars Werkö asked Lars Carlson about differences in the triglycerides in Stockholm and in the United States.

Lars A. Carlson thought that nowadays the methodology of measurement is no problem unless one considers sampling. Most studies in the States did not use fasting samples but in the Stockholm study fasting triglycerides were measured. Lars Carlson was not surprised about differences between the United States and Europe and would say, why should this not be so? What is true in Heidelberg does not need to be true in Jena so why should the circumstances in the United States be the same as in Europe? The panel had already discussed differences in mortality rates and the fact that Ancel Keys' beautiful equation does not fit all the time. He thought it is important not to generalize from one part of the world to another. This may be also true concerning generalizing from Göteborg to all of Sweden.

In regard to the question about the relationship between hypertriglyceridemia and hyperglycemia or to glucose tolerance *Lars Carlson* could give no answers from his study. He thought these are a very important and interesting questions. He had not studied glucose tolerance. The second question was concerning hypertriglyceridemia and high blood pressure. He was a bit surprised at mention of the correlation between these two variables. In the Stockholm Study he considered that there is almost no correlation.

Geoffrey Rose added a small point in response to Dr Carlson. In one study in London—and he was careful not to generalize to Stockholm—a high correlation was found between fasting serum triglycerides and glucose tolerance in men of all ages and in women after the menopause, but not in women before the menopause.

Ancel Keys had a question for Dr Carlson. How did he handle the matter of the age trend? There is an age trend both in triglycerides and cholesterol and Dr Carlson gave us a median split. What happens when age is considered?

Lars A. Carlson replied that age was considered, the study group being split into different decades of age or even smaller age ranges of the population.

At this point *Lars Werkö* proposed to discuss Dr Tibblin's data particularly the indication that these risk factors are not only risk factors for myocardial infarction, but also risk factors for early death. In fact last year Jerry Stamler showed an interesting trend. Lars Werkö had just recalculated Dr Stamler's last figures and there was a trend for all deaths and for non-cardiovascular deaths to be related to the risk factors. With no risk factor the rate was seventeen and with three risk factors the rate was sixty-seven.

Jerry Stamler said that at this Symposium he had not presented any data on total cardiovascular mortality. What was published in the Inter-Society Commission paper was only coronary mortality. His recollection for the record was that in the pooling project the type of association Gösta Tibblin described was not observed. Tavia Gordon of the National Heart Institute had been extremely interested in this question and had been checking study after study and Dr Stamler understands that, except in his own study in Chicago where some association was indicated, none of the other studies showed any association between serum cholesterol and non-cardiovascular deaths.

Lars Werkö asked his British colleagues to comment on his question.

Jerry Morris said that his group had been working on the data in relation to blood cholesterol but no clear relationship was seen. He cautioned also about the danger of trying to answer this major biological question with too few data.

Gösta Tibblin commented that one difference between the Gotheburg study and other studies is that all the Gothenburg men are of the same age and he thought that it is very difficult to standardize for age concerning causes of death.

Lars Werkö said that the title of the panel was "Risk factors, cause or effect" and that there is an "*X*-factor" that could not be identified. What about the other risk factors? Smoking could well be a causal factor, hypertension also a causal factor. What about blood lipids? Are they causal factors for developing premature death?

Jerry Stamler said he would like to make a philosophical remark, encouraged by what Dr Carlson said earlier. He thought that the prospective method can be very useful in special circumstances testing hypotheses concerning causation. Precisely because it is descriptive and not a controlled experiment one is always left with some degree of uncertainty. To go more deeply into cause it is necessary to look at the results of other methodology. To Dr Stamler the animal experimental data on changing the diet of rabbits and chickens, of dogs and rats and of most importance of primates, with the resulting changes in serum lipids and the production of lesions, is the most powerful support of the notion that the diet-lipid chain for events is causative. In support of the conclusion from international epidemiology indicating causation one has to judge from the totality of the data. Ultimately, controlled trials are wanted but even after a successful trial it will be desirable to monitor the whole population at large. The best example to consider is, of course, polio vaccination. First there was a trial of mass application and then the follow-up showed a radical change in the total occurrence of the disease. It was hoped in the next few years to follow this sequence with hypertension and with multiple factor intervention in coronary heart disease.

Jerry Morris said that one factor had not been mentioned. He referred to Professor Duguid and his great emphasis on the thrombotic factor in these conditions. So far in epidemiological work very little has been done about this. Rather elementary studies had been done on fibrinolytic activity in African populations and they show quite striking differences. The rather important relationship between fibrinolytic activity and emotional stress and physical activity should be noted. Also there is a suggested relationship between fibrinolytic activity and serum cholesterol. Could this be an X-factor?

Lars Werkö asked whether the situation here is not the same as prevails in regard to psychosocial factors. So far the tools for study are lacking.

Part II
Changing risk factors

Chairman: *Gunnar Biörck*

Lipid reduction by diet

By Paul Leren

It is of course needless to repeat that all these risk factors or association factors rather, not necessarily are causal factors. I think we all begin to feel a little embarrassed by all these factors, and I agree with Irvine Page when he a couple of years ago stated that we now have got enough risk factors, and that sufficient cholesterol and fats have been fed to animals and man. What we now need are intervention studies, good intervention studies.

Personally, I am also a little tired by going around singing the same old songs. May be that is the reason why I hesitate to start on my actual topic —Lipid reduction by diet.

Numerous experimental studies have demonstrated that the cholesterol level can be influenced by dietary manipulations. Kinsell (1952) and Groen (1952) first observed the cholesterol lowering effect of vegetable oils rich in polyunsaturated acids, especially linoleic acid. Later it has been shown that marine oils rich in polyunsaturated fatty acids with 5–6 double bonds also possess a cholesterol lowering effect (Ahrens 1959 with menhaden oil—Nicolaysen 1959 with cod liver oil). Saturated fatty acids increase blood cholesterol. However, the effect seems to be limited to fatty acids with 12, 14 and 16 carbonatoms. Earlier it was thought that dietary cholesterol had no effect on the blood level. It has now been stated that dietary cholesterol has a small but certain increasing effect on the blood level. From changes in serum cholesterol induced by various changes in dietary fats Keys et al. and Hegsted et al. have derived multiple regression equations which can be used to predict the effect on the serum cholesterol level from changes in dietary fats. There is a close correlation between predicted and observed cholesterol changes.

Prospective and epidemiologic studies suggest that atherosclerotic disease can be prevented by lowering blood lipids. During the last 10–15 years several diet studies have been published. They have all aimed at cholesterol reduction only. With regard to triglycerides no clinical controlled dietary trial has yet been performed aiming at the effect of a reduction of the triglycerides as such. However, conventional cholesterol lowering diet, substituting polyunsaturates for saturated fats, will also have a reducing effect on the triglycerides as demonstrated in my diet study and in the American National Diet Heart Study.

The dietary studies have been undertaken both with subjects free of clinical disease (primary prevention trials) and with patients having survived a heart attack (secondary prevention trials).

The secondary trials are in many ways easier to manage because survivors of a myocardial infarction usually are more motivated for diet restrictions than healthy people. However, the use of patients in such studies involves certain drawbacks, because a negative result may be interpreted in two ways. The treatment may be judged generally ineffective or to be ineffective because the trial was undertaken in subjects with advanced atherosclerosis in whom other factors than an elevated blood lipid level might have assumed greater prognostic significance.

Let us start with the primary prevention studies. All of them used a substituted fat diet with liberal amounts of polyunsaturated fats. All these studies showed a beneficial effect on atherosclerotic disease incidence from the change of diet. Critics can be raised with regard to the design of the Anticoronary Club Study in New York and also of the Finish study, both omitting proper randomization of their study groups. However, Turpeinen and his group have partly made up for this by making a switch over of the study hospitals after 6 years, so that the previous experimental hospital became a control hospital and vise verca. Turpeinen recently on an international atherosclerosis congress in Toronto presented his new data. They are most promising. First, the lipid values were now reversed and with regard to new CHD events after 4–5 years, there is a definite trend towards a lower CHD incidence in the new experimental hospital.

The Dayton study in Los Angeles also deserves special attention. It is the first dietary study based on the double blind principle. It resulted in a reduced cardiovascular morbidity and mortality in the dietary managed group. However, total mortality was the same in both groups, mainly due to an increased cancer mortality in the diet group. We might return to this cancer question in the discussion. Now, I would just like to remind you that in the senium cancer death in fact is almost the only alternative to a death from atherosclerotic disease. The Dayton study is often characterized as a primary prevention study. However, I think you all will agree that one can not talk of primary atherosclerosis prevention at the age of 66, the range being 55–89 at the start of the trial. Moreover, examination at entry positively revealed possible or definite CHD in 1/3 and cerebral and peripheral atherosclerotic complications in many others.

Then, let us take a look at the secondary prevention studies. Some of these studies are not considered of adequate construction suffering from faulty design and dealing with small numbers of patients. I will not review all these studies. The number of trials that have demonstrated positive or improved results with dietary measures is suggestive of a beneficial effect of cholesterol reduction.

With professor Morris present, it might be of special interest to discuss two of the secondary studies more closely, the London study of the Morris group and the Oslo study which I conducted, and try explain why the these seemingly similar studies gave different results. This comparison refers to the first 5-year phase of the Oslo study. The numbers at start are very much the same in both studies. However, whereas each man was followed for exactly five years in the Oslo study, only 90 were left in the London study after 5 years. The most important points are difference in time from primary infarct to entry in the study, the different numbers of hypertensive subjects included, the difference in cholesterol levels, and the difference in time of exposure, the latter being some 30 % shorter in the London study.

In Oslo, the study period started 1–2 years—in average 20 months—after the infarct, in London immediately following the hospital stay. Thus, the London study include the higher recurrence rate during the first year after a myocardial infaction. On the other hand, in Oslo the cholesterol start level was higher than in London—296 and 272 and the Oslo study included distinct hypertensives, 43 % vs. 12 with diastolic blood pressure above 100 mm Hg.

The number of man/years of exposure was higher in Oslo, and the achieved cholesterol difference between the experimental groups is also higher in Oslo. Fatal CHD relapse thus occurred in 37 and 50 in Oslo and in 25 in both groups in London. There was a significant difference in thc major CHD relapse incidence in favour of the diet group in Oslo, but only a trend in London. The numbers of total cardiovascular deaths were 38 and 52 in Oslo and 27 and 25 in London. It is interesting to notice that the relative cardiovascular deathrates are the same in the Oslo diet group and in both the London groups, whereas it is distinctly higher in the Oslo control group. It is natural to attribute this higher deathrate in the Oslo control group to its higher cholesterol level.

I would now like to present the results of the continued follow-up of the men in the Oslo Study.

Clinical and laboratory examinations of the men were discontinued when each man had stayed in the trial for exactly five years, as was diet instruction in the diet group. At the end of this 5-year period the surviving dieters were advised to adhere to the cholesterol lowering diet in the future. The death incidence at the point when the last man to enter the study had stayed in it for exactly 10 years will be presented. At his point 3/4 of the survivors had been in the trial for 11 years. No person in the original groups has been lost to follow-up. There is no significant difference between the groups in overall mortality. The overall sudden death incidence is the same in the two groups. Fatal myocardial infarction occurred in 32 dieters and 57 controls. This difference is highly significant. The total CHD deaths (fatal myocardial infarction+sudden death) were 79 in the diet group and 94 in the control group. This difference is not significant on the 5 per cent level, nor is the total cardiovascular mortality significantly different in the two groups. The mortality rates have been calculated by the Life Table Method taking into account the number at risk in the various years of the trial. There was a higher death rate from myocardial infarction in the control group. The difference is small during the two first years of the trial. The curves for total CHD deaths demonstrates the same trend, although the differences between the groups are statistically not significant at the five per cent level.

The overall survival rates showed only a small difference between the groups.

At the age <60 the patients who died of CHD have a higher mean cholesterol value than the survivors. The difference is highly significant ($P=.01$, both groups combined). At the age >60 there is no such difference.

The importance of combined risk factors in post-myocardial patients was also evaluated. In both groups combined, the CHD mortality rate is 3 times higher in the hypertensive smokers with a cholesterol level above 250 compared with the normotensive non-smokers with a cholesterol level below 250. This difference is also highly significant ($P=.007$).

Also special lipoprotein patterns as first demonstrated by Gofman and revived and extended by the Fredrickson group, have been related to CHD. It is possible that this approach might prove to be more adequate than the study of the isolated blood lipids. However, to my knowledge, no diet intervention studies exist relating the incidence of CHD to the Fredrickson lipoprotein types.

Lipid reduction by drugs

By Per From Hansen

One of the most important measures in preventive cardiology is reduction of the serum lipids, either by dietary means or by drugs, especially focused on high risk groups.

The effect of diet is rather well established, at least on serum cholesterol, as it has been expressed in the equations of Keys and others.

Very little is known, however, about the average effect of various drugs in hyperlipidemic population groups and about the effect of one drug compared with another, expressed quantitatively. Also, very little is known about the combined effects of drugs.

Very many drugs are at the moment available for preventive treatment, e.g. thyroid hormones, clofibrate, nicotinic acid and derivatives and resins. The frequency of side effects by using these drugs seem to be reasonably low.

These many drugs act by different mechanisms and act on different sites in the organism. Therefore, combinations of drugs might possibly exert an increased lipid lowering effect, surpassing that of any of the drugs given alone. Here again, very little has been published about the effect of combined therapy, expressed quantitatively.

In order to try to establish a quantitative evaluation of the lipid lowering drugs available, a nine weeks trial was performed repeatedly in a number of patients with hyperlipidemia, preferably hypercholesterolemia.

The first 6 weeks of each course was a treatment period, through which the reduction in serum lipids was determined, and the subsequent 3 weeks were free of treatment.

It is commonly agreed that the full serum lipid lowering effect of a drug is obtained in not later than 5 weeks, and it can be expected that the effect has subsided and initial values regained after subsequent 3 weeks free of treatment.

The serum cholesterol values 3 weeks after termination of a treatment course do not differ from the values obtained after a longer intermission.

Important for a standardized trial as the one described here is the reproducibility.

Figure 1 and 2 shows the serum cholesterol and fasting triglyceride value respectively after repeated series of treatment with the same drug (clofibrate). The reproducibility seems to be fairly good.

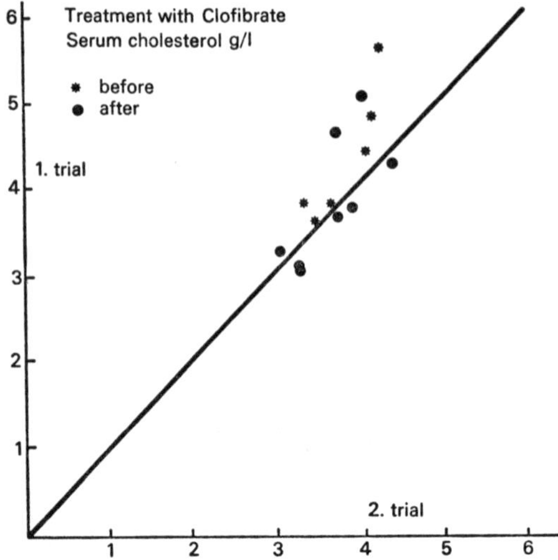

Fig. 1. Serum cholesterol values in seven patients before and after two treatment courses of six weeks duration with clofibrate.

The sensitivity was great enough to show a dose response relationship after treatment with Bufor (*R*) Perycit (*R*) on two dose levels.

The findings here demonstrated seem to indicate that a procedure like the one described meets the requirements for a simple, though sensitive, repeatable and reproducible test, thus creating the possibility for testing various drugs and minimizing the interindividual variability by allowing repeated tests in the same subject.

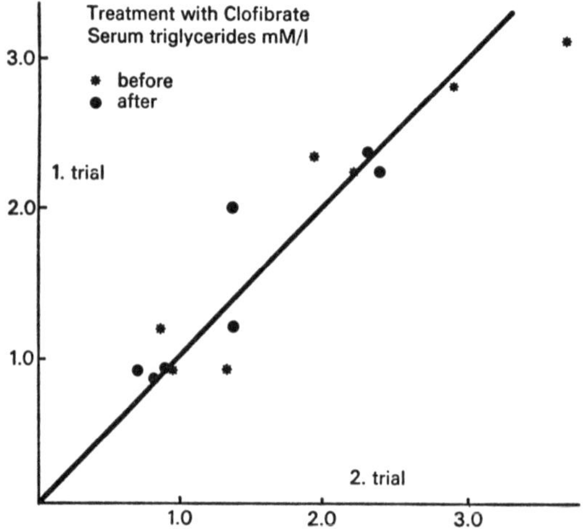

Fig. 2. Fasting serum triglyceride values in the same seven patients before and after two treatment courses of six weeks duration with clofibrate.

Drug	Daily dose	Series no.	Serum cholesterol in g/l before	after	Reduction abs.	%
Clofibrate	2–2.5 g	141	4.25	3.65	0.60±0.06	14
l-thyroxin	0.2 mg	40	4.19	3.72	0.47±0.06	11
d-thyroxin	6 mg	72	3.99	3.47	0.52±0.07	13
Bufor	3 g	25	3.89	3.29	0.60±0.08	16
Cuemid	12 g	23	4.02	3.49	0.53±0.05	13
Clof. + l-thyr.		18	4.32	3.41	0.91±0.17	21
Clof. + d-thyr.		15	4.51	3.39	1.12±0.14	25
Clof. + Bufor		11	3.75	2.71	1.04±0.13	28
Clof. + Bufor + Cuemid		6	3.67	2.78	0.88±0.22	24

Drug	Daily dose	Series no.	Serum triglycerides in mM/l before	after	Reduction abs.	%
Clofibrate	2–2.5 g	51	1.46	1.19	0.27±0.06	18
l-thyroxin	0.2 mg	36	1.33	1.29	0.04±0.08	3
d-thyroxin	6 mg	16	1.26	1.17	0.09±0.09	7
Bufor	3 g	24	1.46	1.14	0.32±0.14	22
Cuemid	12 g	22	1.45	1.47	−0.01±0.04	0
Clof. + l-thyr.		14	1.24	1.03	0.21±0.08	17
Clof. + d-thyr.		11	0.94	0.77	0.17±0.08	18
Clof. + Bufor		11	1.27	0.80	0.47±0.11	37
Clof. + Bufor + Cuemid		6	1.49	1.10	0.39±0.24	26

Fig. 3 and 4. Average serum cholesterol and fasting triglyceride values before and after repeated treatment courses with various drugs given alone and in combination.

	Serum cholesterol in g/l <3	3–3.9	4–4.9	5+
Clofibr.				
before	0	9	4	2
after	4	5	4	2
Bufor				
before	0	8	6	1
after	4	8	2	1
Clof. + Bufor				
before	1	9	4	1
after	10	2	3	

Fig. 5. Serum cholesterol values in 15 patients before and after treatment courses with clofibrate, Bufor and clofibrate+Bufor respectively.

Results

Figure 3 and 4 show the serum lipid lowering effect of various drugs estimated by the above mentioned technique.

The figures indicate that combination of certain pharmaca–especially clofibrate and Bufor –produces a stronger effect than either drug administered alone. The reduction obtained by combined therapy is capable of taking even pronounced hypercholesterolemic values down into the normal range as seen in Figure 5.

Objections against using a combined treatment could be raised because of fear of drug interaction. In the present series nothing has been observed which could be interpreted as increased frequency or severity of side effects.

On the contrary, one should rather expect that drugs acting on different locations or by different mechanisms, in stead of imposing heavily upon one single metabolic process by increasing the dose of a single drug, may reduce the risk of side effects.

Conclusion

Drug combination seems to be a more efficient serum lipid lowering procedure than treatment with any single drug and should be taken into consideration in individual cases of severe hyperlipidemia and in treatment of high risk population groups as well.

Supported by grants from The Danish State Research Foundation, The Danish Heart Association and Cold Stores' Foundation.

Antihypertensive treatment and myocardial infarction

By Bertil Hood

Three sets of data will be brought forward for discussion.

1. Analysis of the four major causes of death in consecutive cohorts of severe hospital-admitted hypertensives. Five and ten year mortality figures.
2. Inter-relations between blood pressure, serum-cholesterol and triglyceride in myocardial infarction occurring at an early age – $\leqslant$50 year.
3. Quantitative aspects of the therapeutic problem. Cut-off points. Coordination-specialists-practitioners.

A material of 1 260 severe hypertensives admitted into two University Departments of Internal Medicine between Okt. 1th 1950 to Dec. 31th 1962 and followed through to the end of 1969 has been divided into consecutive series according to the period in which treatment was started. Analysis of ten year mortality necessitated re-forming of these series, which is the reason why the series covered different periods of time in the ten – as compared with the five year mortality analysis.

There is a very definite difference in our material compared with the other big material started at about the same time (1950) – that of Smirk and co-workers from New Zealand. While Smirk and co-workers excluded those patients, who due to long distances, neglect etc. went out from under their direct supervision, we have on the other hand included all where active treatment had been started with the one single reservation that if surviving the hospital stay the patients should have turned up for one single visit after becoming ambulatory. Early deaths during the hospital stay were included.

A considerable part of the material was sent to practitioners and other specialists in internal medicine etc.

Thus the team of specialists interested in hypertension were in continuous charge of only about 60–65 per cent of our material.

Earlier analysis of our own 1963 and 1965 showed a) that whereas the vast majority of those who suffered letal cerebravascular lesions were to be found among those who were classed as outright failures of control or had entirely gone out of treatment one half of the letal myocardial infarctions had control classed as good or excellent for a considerable period

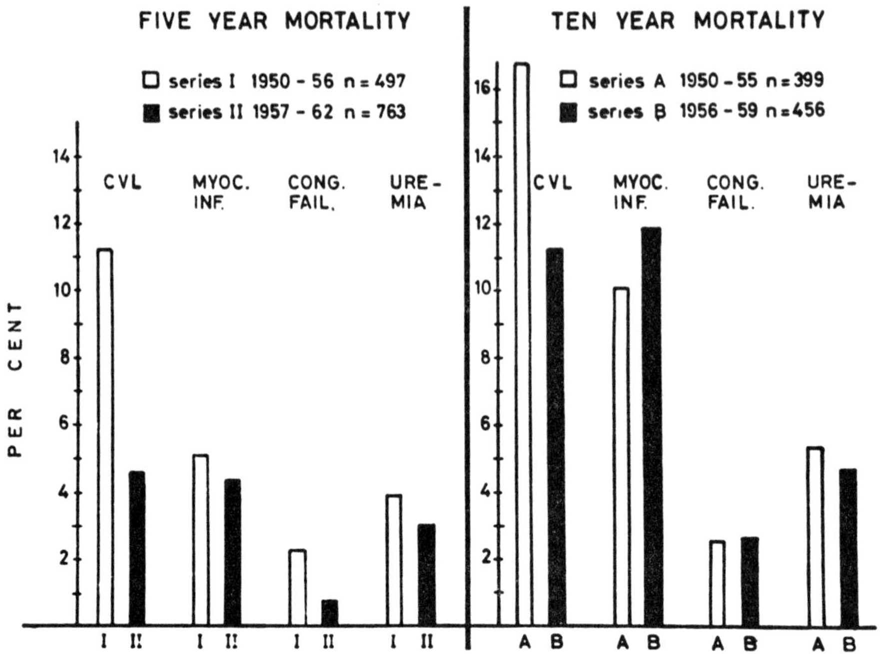

Fig. 1. Left part–five year mortality in severe hospital-admitted hypertensives in the four major causes of death. Two consecutive series.
Right part–the corresponding 10 year mortality.
Caution: The two consecutive series have been re-formed and cover slightly different years.

prior to the attack. In agreement with this myocardial infarction rapidly became the outstanding cause of death in Smirk and co-workers material where patients escaping from their supervision were excluded from material, whereas cerebrovascular lesions still appear as the largest cause of death in our material. The relative proportion of myocardial infarction is definitely on the increase, as the other causes of death diminish in importance. This seems to be most readily apparent in the recent work of Zacharias and co-workers. This recent study covered 325 patients in a five year study; there were 16 deaths, ten of which were due to myocardial infarction.

Deaths due to uremia occurred fairly early after start of treatment (the great majority in 3 months to a year), letal cerebrovascular lesions had a fairly sharp peak in the second year after initiation of treatment in our material.

In contrast to this the letal myocardial infarctions did occur at a steady low rate throughout the entire course of observation. There was no signs of a peak, particularly not in the early period of treatment, not even in the early part of the fifties, when the use of ganglionic blockers not infrequently produced prolonged episodes of hypotension.

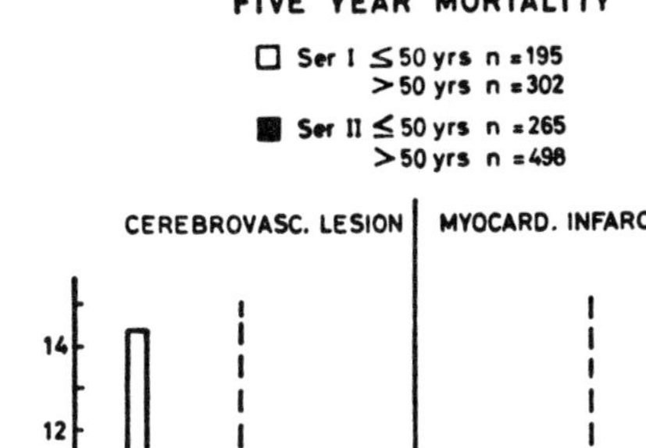

Fig. 2. Five year mortality in cerebrovascular lesions and myocardial infarctions. Material subdivided according to age 50 and 50 at start of treatment.

An analysis of the 5 year mortality of the four major causes of death 1965 in three successive cohorts, taken into treatment in the early, middle and late fifties showed a virtual disappearence of congestiv failure, a sharp reduction of uremia and a 50 per cent drop of deaths due to cerebrovascular lesions. In contrast to this the five year death rates of myocardial infarction remained absolutely stable around 5 per cent in all the three successive cohorts.

Larger material and prolonged times of observation have made possible a recent analysis to evaluate both five and ten year mortality in two successive cohorts. As seen in the right part of the diagram the ten year analysis still showed some improvement in the second as compared with the first series as regards cerebrovascular lesions. There was no such difference, however, in the other causes of death. Also the ten year mortality rate of myocardial infarction was somewhat more than twice as high as the one at five years, again suggesting a very steady rate of occurrence of letal myocardial infarctions throughout the period of active treatment. Fig. 1.

Subdividing the material (Fig. 2) in those ⩽50 and >50 at the start of treatment and looking at five year mortality from cerebrovascular

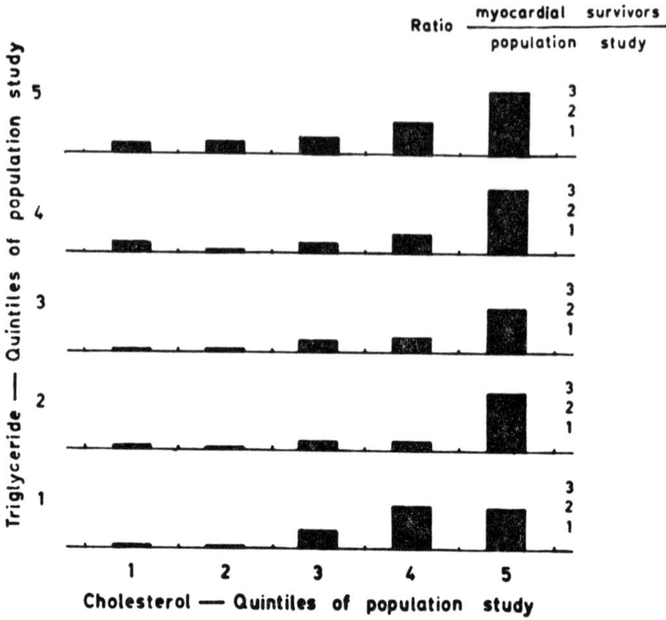

Fig. 3. Ratios myocardial survivors / population study group within each quintile as defined by the population group. Serum cholesterol and serum triglyceride.

lesions the improved result in the second cohort (end of the fifties–beginning of the sixties) as compared with the first looks dramatic for those below the age of 50, while still very demonstrable for those above 50.

As regards myocardial infarction there seems to be an improvement in the second cohort only for those below the age of 50 at start of treatment. The deaths were few, however, and the material in the second cohort below 50 numbered only 265 individuals. It seems vise to refrain from highflying statistics and interpretations. Thus, it seems as if death rates of myocardial infarction were lagely uninfluenced in clinical materials of treated hypertensives. As other causes of death decline the relative role of myocardial infarction becomes greater.

The second problem formulated in the introduction was to try to analyse interrelations between cholesterol, triglyceride and blood pressure. 230 myocardial survivors, all having acquired their first myocardial infarction at or below the age of 50 were compared with a random material of exactly 50 years old males from the same area (the material of Tibblin and coworkers). After correcting for the different size of the two materials, ratios for myocardial survivors/random population study group were then

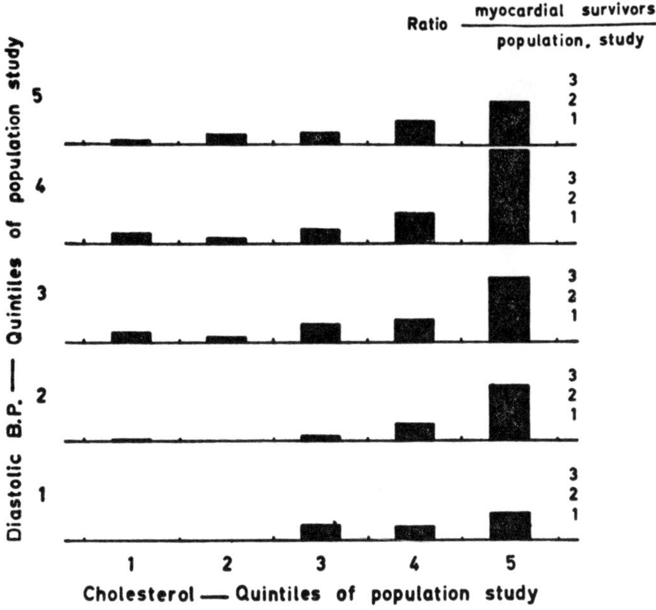

Fig. 4. Ratios myocardial survivors / population study group within each quintile as defined by the population group–serum cholesterol–diastolic blood pressure.

formed for each quintile as defined from the population group of cholesterol, triglyceride and blood pressure respectively.

Let us to familiarize you with the diagram first turn to the one (Fig. 3) showing relations cholesterol-triglyceride. The high ratio myocardial infarction survivors/population group in the two and particularly the highest quintile for cholesterol is easily seen. When triglyceride was high but cholesterol within the two lowest quintiles the ratios were clearly below 1.0, in other words myocardial survivors were underrepresented in relation to the population group.

Fig. 4 then, pictures the relation cholesterol–diastolic bloodpressure. On the whole it gives a somewhat similar idea as the preceeding fig. High ratios in the highest quintile for cholesterol. Here, however, in the bottom right hand corner, the ratio was somewhat less than 1.0. This would in other words mean that myocardial survivors with serum-cholesterol in the highest and a diastolic blood pressure in the lowest quintile were somewhat underrepresented as compared with the population group.

Ratios in the top left corner was very low–in other words there were very few myocardial survivors with high blood pressure and low cholesterol. Myocardial survivors with both serum cholesterol and diastolic blood pressure in the two lowest quintiles did for practical purposes not exist.

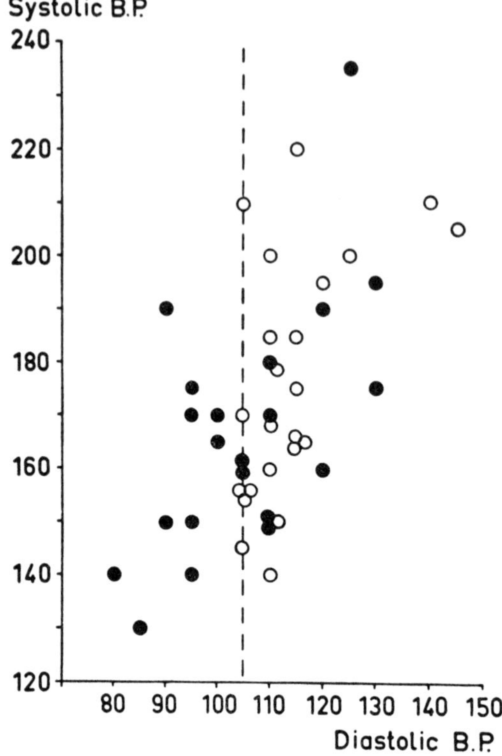

Fig. 5. Distribution of systolic and diastolic blood pressure in a male population, 50 years of age, when a diastolic blood pressure of 105 or known treated hypertension were used as criteria for inclusion in the diagram. Open symbols untreated. Filled in symbols treated.

These are only some of the many observations which might be put forward to argue the existence of a definite hierarchy among the risk factors. The data in this regard might also be conceived of as an argument for a very strict degree of control ideed–pushing the diastolic levels below 80–85 mm.

The third problem concerns how we are going to handle the quantitative aspects of first class blood pressure control if we are going to induce control on liberal indications and at low cut off-points. The very much discussed Veterans Administration Cooperative Study would seem to argue in such a direction.

We have started a study in preventive medicine. We have definitely not limited ourselves to preventive cardiology. We think that the term preventive cardiology should be omitted for a number of reasons. This is a rather intense type of thing–submitting about 30–35 per cent of screened middle-aged males to further work-up and some 25–30 per cent to active

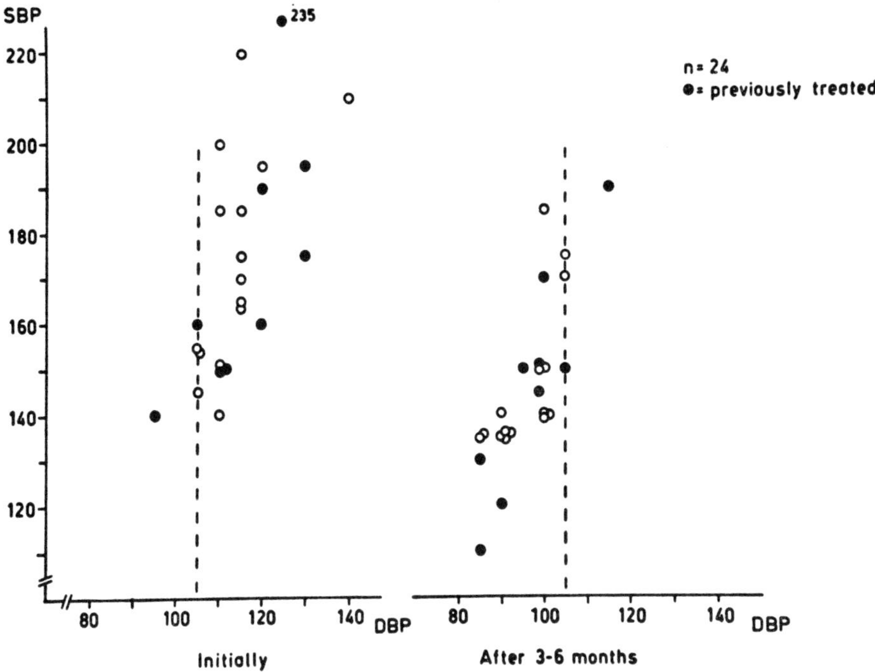

Fig. 6. Symbols same as in fig. 5. Left: Initial distribution of blood pressure. Right: Distribution of blood pressure after 3–6 months on treatment.

measures of various kinds. We are insisting on the highest possible degree of control of serum lipids, chemical diabetes and blood pressure. Hypercalcemia and a number of other findings are carefully worked up. All this is mentioned to show that a) initial rate of screening must adapt itself to the magnitude of the resources for work-up and chronic control, b) all chronic control but in complicated situations must after control has been initiated by a group of specialist teams be transferred to the care of practitioners, practising specialists of internal medicine and health officers. In the Uppsala area these have been submitted to a rather intense program of postgraduate education with particular emphasis on atherosclerosis, diabetes and hypertension. A rather simple computerized system of surveillance has been agreed upon. Using a cut off-point of 105 diastolically and including known hypertensives on drugs presenting levels below this figure the total figure has up till now been 8 per cent in the new 800 screened 49 and 50 year old males. These would according to the stipulations above require chronic control. We are in the beginning of this work; only 800 have been screened and thus about 250–300 actively taken care of in various ways. Resources are, however, gradually increasing and the

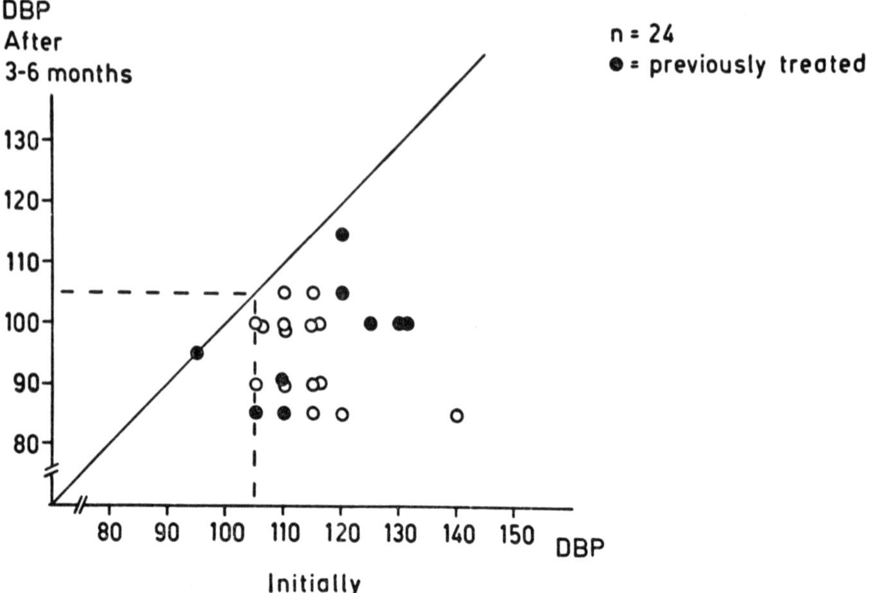

Fig. 7. Diastolic blood pressure. Initially versus at 3–6 months on treatment. Symbols same as in fig. 5 and 6.

screening rate will probably be stepped up. A few preliminary data on blood pressure in the first subsample are given in Figures 5–7.

The initial distribution of systolic and diastolic levels in previously untreated (open) and treated (filled-in symboles) show that a not inconsiderable number were well controlled before our investigation but that also some previously unknown with diastolic levels ⩾130 and above and were found.

Those at or above 105 mmHg diastolic were then within 3–6 months brought under control and very extensively instructed (Fig. 6 and 7). We used propanolol as the first drug up to a dosage of 1 000 mg, usually 320–480 mg/24 hrs. In a few resistant subjects addition of hydralazin up to 200 mg daily or saluretics in a small dose was necessary to institute control.

The aim of this particular detail in our work is then that a decision should be made between 3 and 6 months whether the subject is a complicated one (extremely severe, borderline renal, severely hyperuricemic, presenting multiple problems – hyperlipidemia, chemical diabetes) and therefore should remain in the hands of the team of specialists. The rest of the patients is randomized and one half sent to other physicians – the aim being to see whether initially good control can be maintained to the same degree in the non-specialist as in the specialist-treated group. If so all but the complicated ones will in the future be transferred.

In the specialist's outpatient office nurses and assistents are trained to take care of all details but crucial instructions and decisions. This has lead to a remarkable step-up in turnower, apparently without loss of efficiency, rather with a gain.

When hypertension is defined as problem no 1 but when other risk factors are present emphasis is from the outset put on a two- or three step procedure where first blood pressure control and then the other problems in successive steps are delt with.

Group instruction sessions have been held both in hyperlipidemic disorders and hypertension with group sizes varying between 2 and 5. It is my personal impression, for the value it may have, that problems differ so much between different subjects that even a very experienced and therapeutically interested physician cannot in an efficient manner cope with a group larger than three individuals. There are too many balls left up in the air. The juggling tends to go out of control. Again we have up till now only discussed the comparatively simple problem of attacking some major conditions in a rough fashion in middle age males. Let us now for a moment assume that some of these opportunities should be given to middle-aged women. Let us then visualize a moderately hypertensive, slightly hypercholesterolaemic lady with a lump in her breast, or 10 000 coli per ml urine or a number of suspect and restless cells in the cervical smear or any combination of all this. Much as the methology of screening and the coordination of differently directed programs is completcly necessary and a complicated and fascinating problem there is to me no question that the crucial and rate-limiting step of any program or programs is the delivery of the information to the individual subjects. They should be taken in the hollow of the hand, really cared for and then be liberated in due time.

This takes a lot of experience.—This experience is not necessarily possessed by all eager young epidemiologists or new proselytes to the preventive field so much an vogue.

Anti-smoking programmes

By Geoffrey Rose

I shall consider only a very few of the many important questions posed by the subject of cessation of smoking and its relation to cardiovascular disease.

1. What effects can be expected when middle-aged men stop smoking?

At the present time we have no direct answer to this question. Even if we proved that cigarette smoking is a direct cause of arterial disease, it would not follow that removal of that cause after 20 years or more of exposure would necessarily brings benefits: it could be too late. Nor, even if it were not too late, could we predict with any confidence the rate at which benefits could be expected to appear. If smoking affects arterial diseases by way of thromboic mechanisms, then benefit from cessation might be immediate. If on the other hands, as perhaps seems more likely (1), the mechanisms is related to atherogenesis, then the benefits of withdrawal might be slower to appear. A good deal of indirect evidence is available to us, arising from those of the prospective studies of smoking that are large enough to examine cardiovascular mortality of ex-smokers according to the interval from withdrawal, and to compare it with the experience of life-long non-smokers on the one hand and continuing smokers on the other. The general pattern emerging from these studies (2, 5, 6) seems to be that the excess CHD mortality of current cigarette smokers greatly decreases after cessation, and that after 5 or 10 years it has largely disappeared.

This is encouraging, but there are one or two difficulties in its interpretation. The first is that those men who decide to give up smoking are not a random sample of the smoking population. Some may be men with a better-than-average expectation of long life and health. Others are certainly (4) men who have stopped smoking as a result of ill health, whose life expectation is much worse than average. This would tend to weight the experience of the ex-smokers' group adversely, and to underestimate the benefits of stopping and the rate at which these benefits appear. Against this there may be a possibility that the men who stopped smoking may at the same time also have made other beneficial changes in their habits—for example, taking more exercise.

A similar indication—encouraging but not conclusive—emerges from a recent analysis of the experience of British doctors (8). Fifteen years ago this group had a reported CHD mortality which was higher than that of the United Kingdom population as a whole (a fact which was generally attributed to the pressures of professional responsibility). Subsequently the doctors' rates have been found to fall, whereas those for the general population have risen. As a result the doctor' rate is now below the national level (a change which is not generally attributed to lessening of the professional burden). This is an encouraging illustration of the possibility for an affluent group to reduce its CHD incidence. The explanation must be speculative; but the most likely interpretation is related to the fact that, of British doctors who smoked cigarettes fifteen years ago, most have now stopped.

A number of those who have stopped cigarettes continue to smoke a pipe or cigars. At present there is inadequate information to indicate the disease experience of this group, but in the meantime it seems wise to be cautious about the benefits of such a change for those who continue to inhale or for those who smoke a large number of small cigars as cigarette-substitutes.

From the results of these various observational studies I personally conclude that the evidence, though not certain, is good enough to justify doctors in advising the public and their patients that abandonment of cigarette smoking—even after 20 years of the habit—is likely to reduce the risk of developing atherosclerotic disease. It needs, however, the results of controlled trials to estimate the size of the benefit and the rate at which it can be expected to appear.

In assessing the results of stopping smoking we must consider not only the benefits but also the adverse effects. Only two seem to be important, namely, psychological difficulties and weight gain. In our experience the former mostly turn out to be much less than the subjects themselves predict; and among those who are successful in stopping smoking, they do not often cause disability for more than two or three weeks. The mental trauma may however be greater and longer-lasting among those who do not succeed in stopping.

The virtual absence of long-term psychological disability among ex-smokers has been confirmed by a recent follow-up study of British doctors (3). The same study also reviewed the weight-gain experience of ex--smokers. It appeared that after stopping smoking the gain averaged 12 lb. (5.5 kg.) but eventually the figure had fallen to 4 lb. (1.8 kg.). Our own ex-

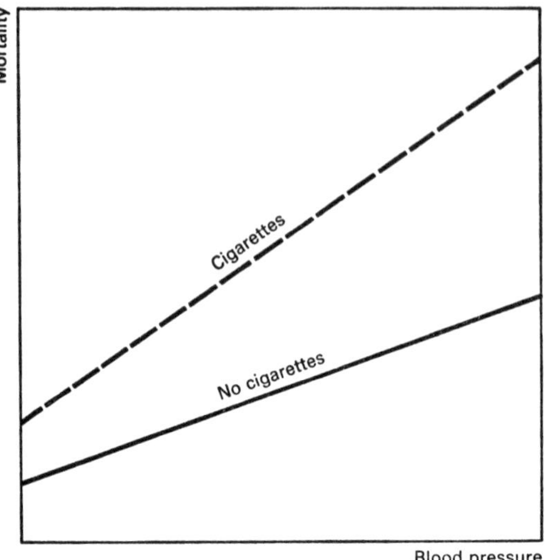

Fig. 1. Schematic representation of the relation between cardiovascular mortality, cigarette smoking, and the level of an independent risk factor (e.g., blood pressure).

perience, with careful early attention to this problem, has been a somewhat smaller average gain at the one-year point. The average figure conceals the fact that among the majority of ex-smokers weight gain is small or absent, but among a few it is a serious problem. The men themselves are often very concerned about this. But as a partial reassurance it can be pointed out that they would probably have to gain an impossibly large amount in order to offset the difference in morbidity and mortality between the ex-smokers and the continuing smokers.

2. Who should be advised to stop?

Ideally everyone should be urged to stop, with the possible exception of those with psychiatric problems and those who are facing exceptional emotional stresses. Resources for giving effective individual advice are, however, limited; hence in practice doctors need to identify those of their patients to whom continued smoking would be particularly hazardous, and who might therefore be expected to gain correspondingly more benefit from stopping.

It turns out (perhaps surprisingly) that cigarette smoking as a risk factor for cardiovascular diseases is largely independent of the other main risk factors: that is to say, the *relative* increase in risk among smokers seems to be approximately the same at all levels of other factors, such as blood pressure and serum cholesterol. This situation is set out schematically in Figure 1, which is based simply on the assumption that at any level of (for example) blood pressure the cardiovascular mortality of cigarette smokers is double that of non-smokers. A simple but important conclusion is apparent from this figure; the *actual* excess risk for the smoker is far from constant at different levels of blood pressure. If we say that at the lowest level the mortality of non-smokers is 1 'unit', then that of the smoker at the same blood pressure level is 2 'units'; the actual cost of smoking at this blood pressure level is then (2–1)=1 'unit'. If we look at the situation for men with high blood pressure, where the mortality of non-smokers is perhaps 4 'units', the mortality among smokers is still doubled, giving them a mortality of 8 'units'; thus the actual cost of smoking at this blood pressure level is (8−4)=4 'units'−4 times greater than for men with low blood pressure.

This leads us to the conclusion that the risks of smoking, the expected benefits from stopping, and hence the importance of giving effective advice, can be enormously more for high-risk than for low-risk individuals. Who are these high-risk individuals, for whom the physician should be constantly on the look-out? So far as cardiovascular diseases are concerned, they are mainly those with a positive family history, those with any elevation (not only those with very high levels) of blood pressure or serum cholesterol, and diabetics. Any of these conditions should at once alert the doctor to the special importance of the smoking problem.

There is another and different reason for concentrating limited resources on high-risk subjects, and that is their greater receptiveness to advice. General statements about statistical risk sound remote to many people until some particular circumstance enables them to accept its relevance to themselves. A clinical diagnosis, or a routine medical examination, may furnish the necessary stimulus. In our experience it has been possible by carefully planned and energetic efforts in high-risk individuals from a cigarette smoking population, to enable more than half of the cigarette smokers to abandon the habit. This level of success seems to be much greater than is commonly achieved in current clinical practice (7).

3. Conclusions

Anti-smoking advice is a preventive and perhaps also a therapeutic weapon of great potential effect. The need is for physicians to recognise its importance, for them to seek more expertise in its application, and for experiment and controlled clinical trials in order to develop more effective methods for its delivery.

References

1. Auerbach, O., Hammond, E. C. & Garfinkel, L.: *New Engl. J. Med 273:* 775, 1965.
2. Doll, R. & Hill, A. B.: *Brit. Med. J. 1:* 1399, 1460, 1964.
3. Fletcher, C. M. & Doll, R.: *Brit. J. Prev. Soc. Med. 23*: 145, 1969.
4. Hammond, E. C. & Garfinkel, L.: *Nat. Cancer Inst. Mono. 19*: 269, 1966.
5. Hammond, E. C. & Horn, D.: *Nat. Cancer Inst. Mono. 19*: 127, 1966.
6. Kahn, H. A.: *Nat. Cancer Inst. Mono. 19*: 1, 1966.
7. Rose, G. & Udechuku, J. C.: *Brit. J. Prev. Soc. Med. 25*: 160, 1971.
8. Royal College of Physicians: *Smoking and health now,* p. 87. Pitman's, London, 1971.

A smoking cessation program in a field trial

By Lars Wilhelmsen

Many people are aware of the health problem caused by tobacco smoking and some want to stop smoking. We have seen a decreased tobacco consumption in Sweden this year, probably because of a fairly intensive propaganda and the percentage of smokers in comparable cohorts studied by us has diminished. Thus in random samples of men examined successively during $1\frac{1}{2}$ years, the percentage of continuing smokers has decreased from 54 per cent in those born in 1915 and 1916 to 49 per cent in those born in 1917. The difference is due to a higher number of ex-smokers in the last cohort.

Smoking has not always been so prevalent as now and nothing indicates that smoking is an essential need for people who have not appropriated the habit.

It is necessary to know the reasons for *continuing* to smoke if you plan to influence the habit. The reasons for beginning to smoke are seldom the same as those for continuing the habit.

Important reasons for continuing to smoke are:

a. One has appropriated a physiological need for nicotine or for the taste of tobacco.
b. Smoking is used to damp anxiety, uneasiness or to increase the level of concentration or it is used for relaxation or to have something in the hand.
c. The "social smoker" smokes because of a tradition in the social environment and may use smoking as an instrument to establish contact.
d. Many smokers who want to stop smoking does not do it because they are afraid of the symptoms following stopping.

Our anti-smoking program has been based on this knowledge and can be divided into four main parts:

a. Measures which increase the motivation to stop. (Most important is information about the health consequences.)
b. Information about the smoking habit. Information about the possibilities to stop does to some extent also influence the motivation.
c. Special withdrawal methods.
d. Supportive treatment after stopping.

The effect of education concerning health consequences and personal experience of symptoms is illustrated by results from our earlier anti-

7 – 729766 *Tibblin m. fl.*

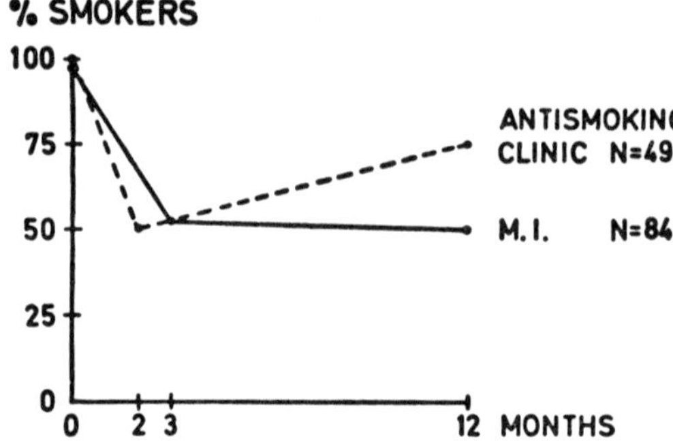

Fig. 1. Percentage of smokers in an anti-smoking clinic (men and women aged 17–65) and in the Post-MI Clinic (men aged 25–57).

smoking work. As is seen from Fig. 1. patients with serious disease or symptoms as after a myocardial infarct (M.I.) stopped smoking and remained non-smokers better than people coming to an ordinary anti-smoking clinic even if the willingness on beforehand was less among the M.I. patients. Much less time was also used in the treatment of the M.I. patients.

Most people do not have definite everyday symptoms referable to smoking. In *primary prevention* the health *consequences* of smoking have to be referred to and little change of the individual condition will be noticed by the subjects themselves when smoking is discontinued. Information bringing about *awareness* of the threat, the individual's *acceptance of the importance* of the threat, the *relevance* of it for the individual himself and susceptibility of the threat to intervention must be of outmost importance. Simultaneously, however, we have to face the possibility of causing mental iatrogenic injuries by our information.

The lack of improvement of the condition in symptomfree individuals is often a serious drawback when we want to increase the motivation. Measurement of i.e. the blood carbon monoxide concentration before and after stopping may be of value as an obvious objective indicator of amount of smoke inhaled.

Smoking is a typical all or none habit for nearly all daily smokers. Very few will be able to cut down their consumption for any considerable time period. A complete and sudden stop is always advised. A relatively short-term, but intensive effort is demanded.

Subjects and methods

In this paper is given our method used in an on-going primary preventive trial comprising 30 000 men in which 10 000 men will be examined and

Table 1. *Anti-smoking schedule in the Preventive Study, Göteborg.*

Meeting	Time	Programme	No. of particip.	Doctor	Psycho-logist
1	0	Inform. about health (consequences and cessation methods)	40	+	+
2	1 week	Cessation method (chewing gum distr.)	7–10	–	+
3	2 weeks	Discuss. of probl. (weight increas., depression etc.)	7–10	+	+
4	6 weeks	Encouraging	7–10	±	+
5	6 months	Encouraging (weight reduction)	7–10	+	+

treated for the risk factors hypertension, high cholesterol and smoking (5). The programme outlined here concerns *all* who smoke 15 grams tobacco a day or more. That is 16 per cent of the sample. We have specially aimed at adopting methods usable in prevention on population basis.

The scedule of the programme is given in Table 1. The first time we invite about 40 persons to an information meeting at which also individual information on results of the earlier examinations is given. A short talk on the health consequences of smoking and the smoking mechanisms introduces a discussion after which the participants are invited to group meetings (7–10 men) with one week's interval for further information about the anti-smoking programme recommended by us and delivery of chewing gum with nicotine. The meetings are conducted by a doctor and one psychologist or other "hostess". This is followed by two to three meetings with one to six months' interval and follow-ups by letters after 3, 6 and 12 months.

Results

The results of anti-smoking treatment may be reconed by different ways; the percentage of subjects who stopped smoking immediately, the per-

Table 2. *Results of anti-smoking programme in the Preventive Study, Göteborg. Cohorts born 1916 and 1917.*

	No.	Per cent
Total number entering the programme	140	100
Stopped smoking at the 3rd meeting	61	44
Reduced consumption to less than 50 per cent	45	32

Table 3. *Results after 2 months with regard to earlier smoking habits in an anti-smoking clinic (Wilhelmsen, 1968).*

	Total no.	Stopped smoking No.	Stopped smoking %	Signif. of diff.
Smoked				
$\leqslant$10 yrs.	56	23	41	$\chi^2 = 4.55$ $p > 0.05$
11–30 yrs.	299	144	48	
>30 yrs.	136	77	57	
Tobacco consumption				
$\leqslant$14 g/day	116	64	55	$\chi^2 = 2.19$ $p > 0.05$
15–24 g/day	278	136	49	
$\geqslant$25 g/day	97	44	45	
Previous attempts to stop smoking	293	93	46	$\chi^2 = 2.09$ $p > 0.05$
No previous attempts to stop smoking	288	151	52	

centage who were still non-smokers after 3, 6 and 12 months and possibly also how many had decreased their consumption or changed over to pipe- or cigarsmoking, but it is naturally also interesting to know to what extent it was possible to prevent disease. Generally, however, we recommend total abstinence as a cut down usually is only temporary.

Today it is only possible for us to give short time follow-up for a sufficient number of people. Table 2 gives the immediate results of the programme.

Table 3 gives some results from an earlier anti-smoking clinic. The number of years smoked, the tobacco consumption or previous attempts to stop had no effect on the outcome. We have made similar findings concerning consumption in our present field trial.

Smoking mechanisms and attitudes

In a field trial it is impossible to give individual councelling and treatment. According to Schwartz and Dubitzky (4) the most commonly offered methods of cessation are the ones least acceptable to smokers, who wish to stop. It is probable that some people should have stopped if our programme had been different.

There is evidence for mainly two types of smokers a) nicotine dependent smokers and b) those where the habituation is more important. In studies performed by Ander et al. (1) it was found, among other things, that those infarct patients who claimed themselves to be nicotine dependent or felt abstinence symptoms when not smoking had a worse outcome of the attempts to stop than others. Even in these persons, however, there is

Table 4. *Results of anti-smoking treatment with chewing gum with nicotine and placebo in the Preventive Study, Göteborg.*

		Doctor 1	Doctor 2	Total
Nicotine	Stopped No.	18	11	29
	Total No.	48	22	70
	Per cent	38	50	41
Placebo	Stopped No.	13	7	20
	Total No.	37	21	58
	Per cent	35	33	34
Total	Stopped No.	31	18	49
	Total No.	85	43	128
	Per cent	36	42	38

usually a fairly strong habituation effect connected with the smoking. The idea with giving chewing gum with nicotine is to supply them with the possible benefits of nicotine in comination with "oral occupational therapy" during a transitional period. We have used chewing gum with nicotine in amounts giving up to the same blood nicotine levels as cigarette smoking and compared the effects with those of placebo chewing gums. The results in a series of persons in the Preventive Study appear in Table 4. As can be seen the difference is small. Other studies and single experiences have, however, given a more positive conception of the effect of nicotine chewing gum. One reason for the difference may be that we, in contrast to others, have delt with persons with moderate troubles to stop. Thus the mean daily consumption of chewing gums was only around 3–4. To show any effect we should probably have used only subjects with evident problems in stopping without the help of nicotine. Thus, our impression is that nicotine is of value in selected cases. It is, however, often seen that people who strongly believe that they are nicotine dependent do only suffer very mild withdrawal symptoms when they stop smoking without nicotine substitution.

In our attempts to improve our anti-smoking methods and possibly to be able to select people for different programmes we have used a translation of an American questionnaire concerning attitudes towards smoking, the dangers of smoking and the motivation for giving up smoking (3). Smokers born in 1917 from the Preventive Study filled in the questions of this at the screening examination. We could not find any item which was correlated to the later outcome of our anti-smoking treatment. The lack of correlation between attitudes towards smoking etc. in this test and the possibilities to stop may be explained by the fact that our information after the test increased their motivation more strongly then their earlier knowledge.

Draw-backs of cessation

Finally, I have to make a short comment on the weight increase which is so commonly seen in those who stop smoking and which sometimes is a reason to begin smoking again. After giving up smoking food tastes better, smells better and besides that people long for something for oral occupation. An increased gastric motility may also be of some importance. All this often leads to heavier meals and taking sweets and similar things between the meals. There are, however, also data speaking for weight increase in spite of no change of caloric intake or physical activity. Single investigations thus indicate a change of metabolism (2). The mean weight increase during the first 2 months uses to be around 2–3 kg:s. At present we have nothing else but caloric restriction and increase of physical excise to offer.

A series of mental problems as nervousness, lack of ability to concentrate, tiredness etc. have been encountered in anti-smoking clinics. Most smokers who stop smoking stop without the aid of special clinics, and it is probable that the clinics see people with more problems at cessation than usual. Our experiences in this field trial support this hypothesis; the number of men with this type of problems has been fairly low.

References

1. Ander, S., Wilhelmsen, L. & Tibblin, G.: Who stops smoking after a myocardial infarction. *Transact. Second Wld Conf. on Smoking and Health,* Sept. 1972.
2. Glauser, S. C., Glauser, E. M., Reidenberg, M. M., Rusy, B. F. & Tallarida, R. J.: Metabolic changes associated with the cessation of cigarette smoking. *Arch. Environ. Health 20*: 377, 1970.
3. Horn, D.: *Smoker's self-testing kit.* U.S. Department of Health, Education, and Welfare, 1969.
4. Schwartz, J. L. & Dubitzky, M.: Expressed willingness of smokers to try 10 smoking withdrawal methods. *Public Health Rep. 82*: 855, 1967.
5. Wilhelmsen, L., Tibblin, G. & Werkö, L.: A unique clinical trial dealing with primary intervention of high risk factors related to myocardial infarction. *Preventive Med. 1:* 1972.

Physical inactivity

By Martti J. Karvonen

Background

Physical inactivity has presented itself as a risk factor for coronary heart disease (CHD) in several epidemiological studies, but not in all of them. In some societies sedentary men have higher *mortality* from CHD than men doing heavy manual work, but the difference does not apply to all countries. It often is, of course, possible that the observed differences in mortality are due to confounding socio-economic variables, such as diet, and not to the degree of physical activity of occupation itself. Competitive sports are a more vigorous form of physical activity than occupational work. Successful participation in endurance skiing has been shown to be associated with a 6 to 7 years higher longevity than that of the corresponding general Finnish male population (1, 2).

Some *prevalence* studies have contributed similar evidence. E.g. electrocardiographic abnormalities characteristic of CHD have been found less frequently among lumberjacks than in other occupations (3). However, such a difference may well be due to bias of selection: it is not likely that men with manifest heart disease would work as lumberjacks, if any other alternatives were open for them.

In longitudinal studies, occupational differences in *incidence* of CHD have not generally been observed. This applies, e.g., to the seven countries' study (4): the physical activity rating, which in these rural populations essentially depended on occupation, did not affect the incidence in any of the cohorts. Leisure-time activity, on the other hand, may have an effect in urban communities. Thus the study by Rosenman et al. (6), best known for its emphasis on personality types as a risk factor, also showed that new cases of CHD occurred significantly more often among those with no exercise habits than among the general population at risk. In the Framingham-study, various indirect indices of physical activity were used to demonstrate that physical activity protects against CHD. One of these indirect measures was vital capacity. A recent analysis by Keys et al. (4) shows that the demonstrated relationship was entirely spurious: with age both vital capacity decreases and the risk of CHD increases, but there was no more direct relation between vital capacity and risk than the association of each with age.

Prevention studies: three generations

In prevention studies, three generations of approach may be observed. A first generation study simply uses man as an experimental animal. Captive populations are preferred as subjects, and the conditions of the study are standardized as far as it is possible. The well-known Finnish dietary prevention trial is a typical example of the first generation studies (10, 11).

The second stage is to attempt prevention among free-living people in their natural environment. Quite a large interdisciplinary team of investitators may be needed and a wide array of research methods used. The 18 months' feasibility study to be reported below belongs to the second generation.

The third, last, generation of prevention studies aims at integrating prevention into the health services; it may also be called a public health experiment. The Göteborg primary prevention program probably could come under this heading.

Why exercise?

Physical activity may be included in a prevention program for two different reasons. First, there are some results suggesting that it may protect against CHD, although the evidence is not nearly as solid as with the primary risk factors, blood pressure, cholesterol and cigarettes. However, physical activity may also be offered to the clients as an acceptable vehicle for other forms of prevention, as a central major change of life, to which other minor changes in habits may easily be added to.

18 months' feasibility study

As an example of a prevention study of the second generation I present a condensed report of a study carried out at the Helsinki Institute of Occupational Health (7, 8, 9, 5). The study had three general purposes:

1. to develop methods of intervention,
2. to measure effects of the training programme, and
3. to form hypotheses concerning confounding variables which may act as modifiers of the effects of the training programme.

The subjects were chosen from men taking part in executive health examinations. The selection of subjects started from 1 345 men, and ended in 89 matched pairs of middle-aged high risk men with either high cholesterol, high blood pressure, or with ischemic ST after exercise. The matching variables were age, serum cholesterol, systolic pressure, ischemic ST depression and smoking.

The testing consisted of fitness measurements every 1.5 months, medical, physical and biochemical studies every three months, and of psychological tests, dietary survey and chest *X*-ray at the beginning and end.

The exercise programme included running, swimming, handball and calisthenics, 45–60 minutes three times a week. The mean participation rate was 72 %, gradually declining from approximately 90 to 60 % of the prescribed number of sessions.

The exercise programme resulted in an increase of 17 % in the predicted aerobic power. There was no effect on body weight, skinfold thickness, serum cholesterol, or on the smoking habits. Blood pressure decreased significantly over 18 months, but just as much in the exercise group as among their controls. In the exercise group, the heart volume and the T-vector increased, but the prevalence of the ST segment depressions was unaffected. Among the psychological variables, significant positive effects were seen in visual speed and in visual concentration. The subjects became less tense, less nervous, their subjective stress tolerance increased, and they found relaxation easier.

The study showed that middle-age Finnish men could be recruited to participate in quite a strenuous programme of supervised training and they adhered to it. Only 12 of the 89 men quitted the exercise programme during 18 months. The programme improved the fitness, but left the other risk factors unaffected.

Third generation plans

Two plans for third generation studies are now maturing in Finland. One of them is to be carried out in Helsinki, in an urban environment. The first step would be a pilot study, building on the experience gained in the 18 months' study. The planning has been done in close cooperation between the City Health and Sport Offices, and the Institute of Occupational Health. Two alternative plans are being considered. The first one consists of screening 4 000 men of 45–54 years of age. Of these 400 high risk men would be selected and divided at random into an intervention group and a control group of equal sizes. The intervention would consist of directed exercise three times a week, plus personal anti-smoking campaign and diet education.

The second alternative appears more ethical. Two thousand men would be screened and another 2 000 controls only picked from the population register. Two hundred high risk men would be subjected to an intense prevention programme, and the remaining 1 800 men would receive a less intense educational programme. A minimum screening would be used, with a follow-up examination after a suitable interval.

The second plan concerns a rural area, Northern Carelia, with the highest mortality from CHD in the entire world. This study should become a real public health experiment applied to the entire population of a county of some 200 000 people, with one or two comparable control areas elsewhere.

Educational spinoff

The studies hitherto conducted have given our group much practical experience in how to organize exercise programs for middle age high risk people. A two weeks' course was offered in August 1971 primarily to municipal sport leaders. The course was fully booked; its material may even find its way into book form.

Summary

Physical inactivity may increase the risk for coronary heart disease (CHD). While the observed occupational differences in risk may largely be due to confounding socio-economic variables, some studies suggest that physically active leisure habits are associated with reduced risk.

Three generations of prevention studies may be carried out. The first preferably uses captive populations under strictly controlled conditions. The second generation is intense studies of free-living people, and the third generation public health experiments.

A completed second generation exercise prevention study and the plans for two third generation studies are described.

References

1. Karvonen, M. J.: Problems of the training of the cardiovascular system. *Ergonomics 2*: 207–215, 1959.
2. Karvonen, M. J., Kihlberg, J., Määttä, J. & Virkajärvi, J.: Longevity of champion skiers. (Finnish with English summary.) *Duodecim 72:* 893–903, 1956.
3. Karvonen, M. J., Rautaharju, P. M., Orma, E., Punsar, S. & Takkunen, J.: Cardiovascular studies on lumberjacks. *J. Occup. Med. 3*: 49–53, 1961.
4. Keys, A., Aravanis, C., Blackburn, H. W., Djordjevic, B. S., Dontas, A. S., Fidanza, F., Karvonen, M. J., Menotti, A. & Taylor, H. L.: Lung function as a risk factor for coronary heart disease. (In press.)

5. Pyörälä, K., Kärävä, R., Punsar, S., Oja, P., Teräslinna, P., Partanen, T., Jääskeläinen, M., Pekkarinen, M.-L. & Koskela, A.: A controlled study of the effects of 18 months' physical training in sedentary middle-aged men with high indexes of risk relative to coronary heart disease. In *Coronary heart disease and physical fitness* (ed. O. André Larsen & R. O. Malmborg), pp. 261–265. Munksgaard, Copenhagen, 1971.
6. Rosenman, R. H., Friedman, M., Strauss, R., Wurm, M., Jenkins, O. & Messinger, H. B.: Coronary heart disease in the Western collaborative group study. *J.A.M.A. 195:* 86–92, 1966.
7. Teräslinna, P. & Partanen, T.: Some characteristics of Helsinki executives in specified age groups: a pilot study aimed at physical activity prophylaxis of coronary heart disease. *Work-Environment-Health 5:* 63–67, 1968.
8. Teräslinna, P., Partanen, T., Pyörälä, K., Punsar, S., Kärävä, R., Oja, p. & Koskela, A.: Feasibility study on physical activity intervention. Report on recruiting design, training program, and three months' experience. *Work-Environment-Health 6:* 24–31, 1969.
9. Teräslinna, P., Partanen, T., Koskela, A. & Oja, P.: Association of certain social habits and attitudes with risk factors of coronary heart disease. *Soc. Sci. Med. 5:* 243–250, 1971.
10. Turpeinen, O., Miettinen, M., Karvonen, M. J., Roine, P., Pekkarinen, M., Lehtosuo, E. J. & Alivirta, P.: Dietary prevention of coronary heart disease: long-term experiment. *Amer. J. Clin. Nutr. 21*: 255–276, 1968.
11. Turpeinen, O., Miettinen, M., Karvonen, M. J., Roine, P., Pekkarinen, M., Lehtosuo, E. J. & Alivirta, P.: Blood lipids and primary coronary events. The effect of diet modification. *Minnesota Med. 52*: 53–58, 1969.

Discussion

Preventive approach to cardiovascular disease–benefits and drawbacks

A discussion on the preventive approach to cardiovascular diseases was opened by the chairman *Gunnar Biörck* who said he had been assigned the role of the devil's advocate and asked to examine what might be the limitations and even drawbacks in the application of the preventive approach. He suggested that this question might be viewed from two standpoints: one that of the gross national product (GNP) and the other "the quality of life".

Gunnar Biörck indicated his belief that the prevention of rubella may prevent some congential heart disease and that penicillin may prevent rheumatic fever and valvular heart disease. But in regard to coronary heart disease and hypertension he thought that the main objective at present can only be the postponement of symptoms, of invalidism and death, and that there the analysis of cost benefit should be made. With a gain of productive years, which contributed to the GNP, there must also be an increase in the years of retirement, which subtracts from the GNP. It was not certain that an economic argument would apply, at least not in Sweden.

Richard Remington's view was that if prevention is attainable, the people will demand it. We and the social planners must decide what to do. In regard to cost, this must be viewed with priorities. Some costs of a screening program could be absorbed by the use of personnel who would otherwise be unemployed.

Gunnar Biörck proposed, because of severe time limits for discussion to move from the economic argument to the question of the quality of life. What can the preventive approach contribute? In order to evaluate that contribution it is necessary to make experiments and carry out trials but at the same time, we must consider undesirable effects. First the diagnostic procedure involves inconvenience, loss of time, loss of earnings, anxiety and pain for the subjects examined. The examination is interference with the "integrity" of the individual. The examination interferes with pre-existing patient-physian relationships. Data obtained in the examination may be disclosed to employers and insurance companies the disadventage to the person examined. Finally the person examined may be lulled into a false sense of security.

Rose Stamler emphasized that prevention is a form of treatment much like therapy for frank disease. It differs in that it is treatment *before* signs and symptoms of the disease appear. And–like other forms of treatment–there are benefits and possible side effects. In looking at benefits and side effects (unfavourable ones), a proper balance is needed, to decide how serious it would be if nothing was done–until the disease appears, after which treatment was started.

Consider coronary heart disease, a disease that affects five and a half million people in the United States. This disease kills 600 000 Americans each year, about one-third of them under 65 years of age. This is the major cause of death in the United States, as it is in many other developed countries in the World. Here is a disease which has a poor response to treatment if nothing is done until the disease is clinically evident. About one in every five heart attacks ends in death within a few hours. One in three or four ends in death within one month. And the "lucky patient" who survives a heart attack is many times more prone to another attack than the person in the same age who has not yet had an attack. This is what must be faced if we sit by and decide to treat only after frank disease is diagnosed. It is against *this* danger that any dangers from a preventive approach must be weighed.

Of course, when any effort is made to deal with large numbers of people and to change some of the things they are doing, new problems must be faced. Look at one question–the effect on the attitude and peace of mind of the man who is examined in a screening program to find coronary risk factors.

What if you find he has hypertension or high serum cholesterol, and is a smoker besides? Wasn't he happier before he learned this? Haven't you upset him? You may have–but if you are able to suggest that there are ways in which he can probably reduce his risk to *normal* risk, and that you can help him do this, you supply a path of positive action for him to compensate for the anxiety.

Would you be doing his peace of mind a better service if you waited until his first heart attack and then, if he survived you tried to reassure him–even though you know his chances of a good life had been greatly reduced?

One would scarely use the arguments proposed by Dr Biörck against detection of early glaucoma, or against the Pap smear. In coronary heart disease early preventive action would seem to be a most effective way of dealing with the problem while waiting for symptoms and frank disease could be and often is fatal.

Do you not rather give a false sense of security if you do not let people know what research has made fairly certain. Should you not let a middle-aged man know that if he smokes a pack or more of cigarettes a day his chance of a coronary event is *three* times that of a man who *never* smoked, and it's two and a half times that of a man who's quit?

Aren't you also obliged to let him know that if his diastolic blood pressure is above 95 mm Hg, he also doubles his chance of a heart attack? And that if his serum cholesterol concentration is 275 mg/100 ml or higher, his susceptibility is tripled.

Of course you would think twice about telling him these things if you could not help him to reduce his risk. But—fortunately—together with helping to clarify risk factors—research, both clinical and epidemiological has indicated that there is a good chance this can be done—in regard to serum cholesterol, hypertension and smoking as risk factors.

A word should be said about possible mistakes in screening for risk factors. You might for example, tell a man he is "normal" while actually he is hypertensive or hypercholesterolemic. Errors of measurement do occur and everything possible should be done to reduce them, but the same kind of errors arise in the individual treatment of the sick patient in a doctors office, in the clinic, in the hospital. In dealing with large numbers of people special care is needed to standardize methods, check for errors, etc. This consideration, however, can not hold us back from the main problem, the huge numbers of true "positives"—who are undetected and untreated, but who can and should be found as the first step of preventive work.

What is said here about coronary heart disease applies as well—perhaps even more—to rheumatic heart disease (a major affliction of millions of young people in the developing countries) and the worldwide afflications of hypertensive heart disease and stroke. To wait until the streptococcus infection leads to rheumatic fever and then to rheumatic heart disease is, clearly the most costly way—in human terms—to go about the problem. No serious inroad into that mass disease can be made without a mass public health approach—both against streptococcus infections and the social conditions of overcrowding, under-nutrition etc., which no doubt help set the stage for this disease.

Henry Blackburn noted that distress, anxiety and loss of income are important determinants of *any* medical procedure, but nowhere in practice or in hospital medicine are they the *primary* factors in medical decisons—when the best medical judgement is that the procedure is indicated. Granted that there have been irresponsible screening program, but there is a much larger experience undertaken by conscientious physicians and investigators, with positive goals, with careful follow-up and evaluation and the information held privileged. In fact, the only "research" screening test done which is not generally available from employment and insurance examination routines is the blood lipid measurement. The argument of trauma to the subject from screening cannot hold as lipid levels are not now grow grounds for any restrictive action in daily life, employment or insurance.

Direct experience in Minneapolis, based on a survey with Dr Taylor of 11 000 homes and their response rate to a carefully prepared and timed screening and preventive program, provides *no* evidence of any serious anxiety, of any unacceptable inconvenience, or any important loss of income. On the contrary, the 90 % response rate, and 100 % approval of treating physicians suggest that the question posed by Prof. Biörck is largely a theoretical one.

Henry Blackburn commented on Gunnar Biörk's worry about possible interference with pre-existing physician-patient relationships. In his experience, the U.S. physician is pleased to have specialized help in patient management and motivation toward hygienic living—as long as the fundamental medical and pharmaceutical management is directed by the physician. In projected trials and community programs which involve direct treatment modes, including therapy for hypertension, hyperlipidemia and hyperglycemia, the overwhelming evidence is that traditional medical care in the U.S. has been inadequate. The methods developed in this current generation of trials and community studies will become freely applicable. In competitive systems, the best method will win and will be adapted and adopted to the medical care delivery system most appropriate and most effective in each case.

In regard to the possible "false security" induced in screened persons by negative findings, it is of interest to look at the usual situation in practice of the overworked U.S. physician: he is unskilled in the evaluation and the modification of future risk and in techniques of health maintenance. After a thoroughgoing, disease-oriented medical examination, at a cost varying from 75 to 1 000, this good physician may have detected a heavy smoker with moderate overweight, some elevation of blood pressure and a cholesterol of 250 mg%. His usual "pat-on-the-back, cut-down-a-bit, take-it-easy, everything-checks-out-O.K." approach is hardly a sound basis for promoting patients security. Findings in a screening program of how the values lie in the total distributions of values for the major risk factors, provide a much more sound basis for promoting patients security.

Finally, in response to the idea that the preventive approach may interfere with the individual's integrity in matters of health, Henry Blackburn thought that "individual integrity in health matters" should be defined. Society is coming to accept medical care and health as an individual's right. We must conclude that with this individual right there is some individual responsibility. If the right of the individual to disable and destroy himself, with the attendant cost to society, is essential to "personal integrity", then society's goals are surely lost.

Gunnar Biörck turned to the aspects of manipulations and saw these possible points unfavourable:

1. Possible side-effects such as a trauma in physical exercise, nervousness during smoking abstinence, toxic effect of lipid, lowering drugs, or ill effects of diet.
2. Still more important may be the anxiety from a new consciousness of hypertension, elevated lipids, the hazard of smoking, etc., particularly if attempts at correction of the risk factors failed to give results or appeared to be unrewarded.

A particularly important question is whether a patient should be informed simply objectively or rather persuaded. What right has the doctor meddling into peoples' ways of life?

Henry Blackburn in reply commented that all methods of treatment have side effects and particularly drugs and surgical treatment in conventional therapeutic medicine. The question is how can these risks be minimized? Clearly the treatment of preventive method recommended should be commensurate with the level of risk, as best we can determined. Generally, the risk from side effects of practising good hygiene, the goal of primary prevention efforts, is not to be compared with the risk of neglect and is not of the same order as risks from drugs or surgery. But, the question is appropriate; for example, the risk of *high level* physical conditioning in grossly sedentary middle-aged men in the U.S. in sufficient that many are recommending only moderate levels of exercise in general, unsupervised prevention programs.

He considered the argument that being conscious of high blood pressure, elevated serum cholesterol, the ill effects of smoking, etc., may create anxiety and this may be even worse if efforts at correcting the "risk factors" fail. He thought it likely that public knowledge of disease risk and modes of reducing the risk is on the contrary the *best* hope, and most logical strategy to reduce the burden of IHD with its much *greater* production of anxiety, inconvenience and loss of income. To keep the population unconscious of the major risk factors of these diseases so that it may nourish the vague hope of one day being struck suddenly dead, hardly provides a basis for sound public health policy.

Henry Blackburn agreed, however, with Gunnar Biörck's suggestion that "prevention" of IHD, if successful, essentially means "postponement", with risks of mortality from other causes competing with cardiovascular disease as the final cause of death. But postponement of death and disability along with relief of pain, is in fact the primary goal of both traditional and preventive medicine, and is what medicine is all about. The fact that the current problems of society among the elderley population are unsolved provides, in itself, no rationale to ignore the challenge of such postponement among those already born on to this overpopulated planet.

Gunnar Biörck said that the final appraisal of benefits and drawbacks depends upon the individual estimate of the qualities in living. He draw attention to the problem of the quality of life. All feel that there may be distinctive gains in happiness and in family cohesion if the father survives until the children are married, so he may happily experience the growth and development of grand children. This may be one of the probable benefits of a preventive program. However, there is one more word to be said. He believed that most people on the one hand want to live for a fairly long time, though perhaps not for a *very* long time. On the other hand those very same people prefer to die a sudden death. How can we prevent sudden death at a younger age and promote it at a later?

Part III
Heart control programme

Chairman: *Jerry Morris*

The WHO heart control programme in Europe

By Z. Pisa

Components of any community control programme directed at any disease include: prevention, detection, treatment including rehabilitation, education and research. A built-in system of evaluation of the impact of any measures introduced under such a programme should nowadays be essential.

Considering the cardiovascular control programmes, the fact is faced that different diseases are involved; the only thing they have in common is that they are affecting the heart and vessels.

Taking also into account the final goals of medical services in most European countries, it should be kept in mind that the general aim of such community cardiovascular disease control programmes should form an essential link in control programmes for chronic diseases in particular and in comprehensive public health programmes in general.

For all these reasons the present attempts of the WHO long-term programme in the field of cardiovascular diseases in the European Region, is to test and evaluate new methods and forms of organization, with a view to developing community cardiovascular disease control programmes integrated in health services in individual countries.

To achieve that, it is necessary first to define the extent of the problem of cardiovascular diseases in the community as precisely as possible, and secondly to see what methods of control are feasible in the present existing situation.

The actual European WHO programme in this field started in 1968. Its first phase planned until 1972 concentrated quite naturally on ischaemic heart disease. Its increasing incidence, especially among younger age groups of males during the last decades is nowadays a recognized fact (Fig. 1, Fig. 2).

The programme proposed included projects dealing with prevention, detection, improvement in the collection of better information on the natural history of ischaemic heart disease in the community, and evaluation of new methods of treatment including rehabilitation. An intensive training programme supported all these activitites. A system of collecting information with the purpose to evaluate the impact of the programme and also to assess its progress is being built up (Fig. 3).

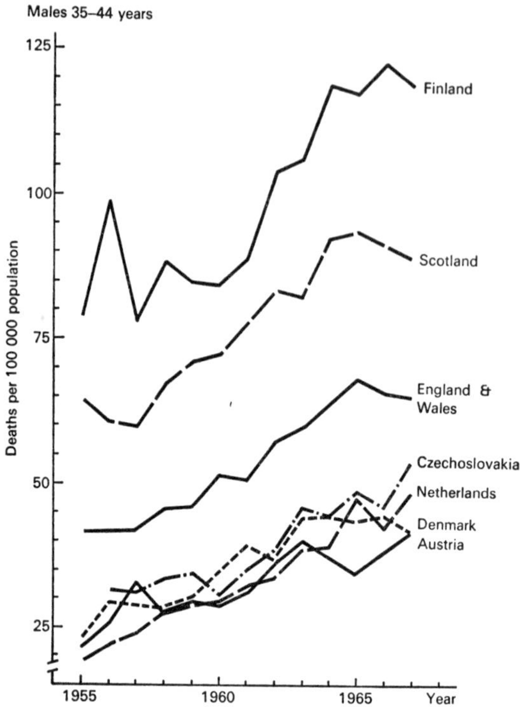

Fig. 1. Age-specific Death rates for ADHD in selected countries 1955–1967.

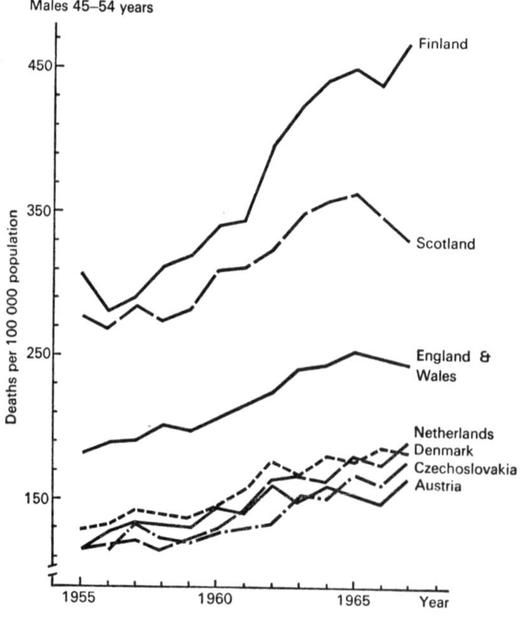

Fig. 2. Age-specific death rates for ADHD in selected countries 1955–1967.

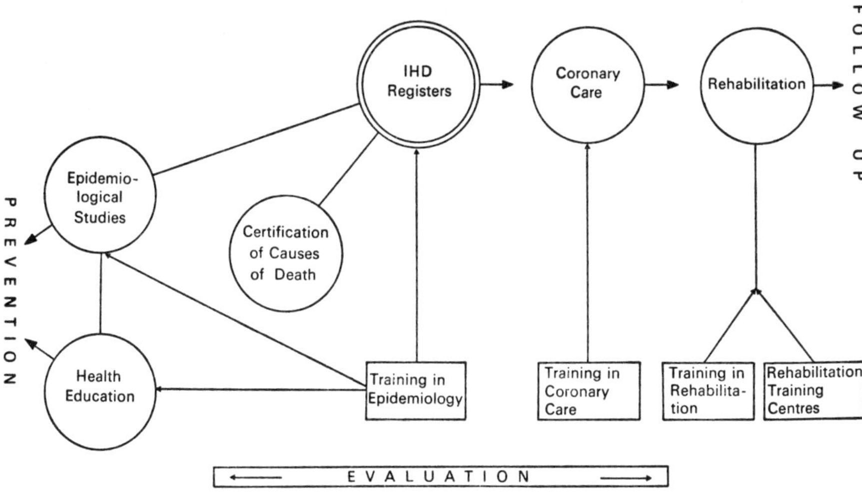

Fig. 3. Euro cardiovascular diseases programme, 1968–1972.

From the very beginning the project on "Establishment of Ischaemic Heart Disease Registers" was considered as a key one. These ischaemic heart disease registers were established on a precisely defined population basis and therefore the information collected reflected reasonably well the situation in each community under study. At present there are 18 of these

Table 1. *Ischaemic heart disease registers.*

Code no.	Country	Pilot area	Population
01	Sweden	Gothenburg	420 000
02	Czechoslovakia	Prague 4	175 000
03	Romania	Bucharest 4	282 276
04	Hungary	Budapest	520 000
05	Denmark	Copenhagen	1 500 000
06	Ireland	Dublin City	142 000
07	Fed. Rep. of Germany	Heidelberg	304 129
08	Finland	Helsinki	540 000
09	United Kingdom	Tower Hamlets London	200 000
10	Netherlands	Nijmegen	230 000
11	Finland	Tampere	155 000
12	Poland	Warsaw	520 000
13	Poland	Lublin	200 000
14	Austria	Innsbruck	157 279
15	USSR	Kaunas	306 000
16	France	Boulogne	
17	Sweden	Boden	40 000
18	Bulgaria	Sofia	237 235 over 19 years 438 334 all ages
30	Australia	Perth	449 969
31	Israel	Jaffa	200 000

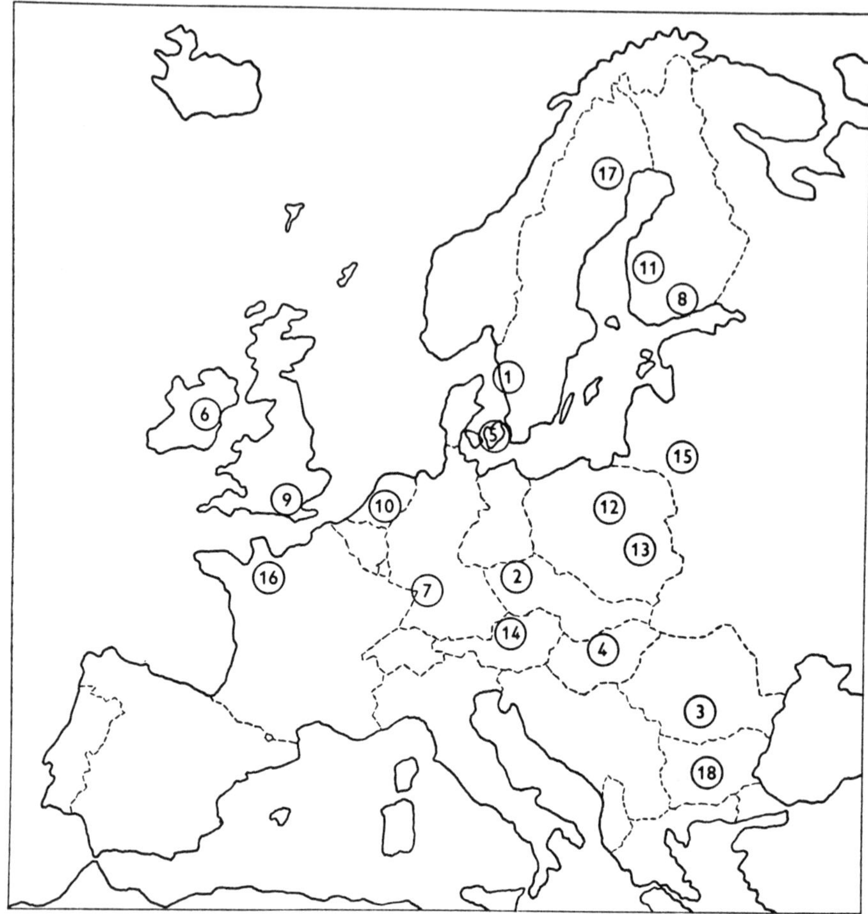

Fig. 4. WHO study: ischaemic heart disease registers in europe (1971).

Populations covered: from 142 000 – Dublin to 540 000 – Helsinki (except Boden – 40 000 Copenhagen – 1 500 000)

registers established and collaborating with WHO in Europe, one in Australia and one in Israel. The population covered is between 40 000 and one and a half million inhabitants, but most of the registers cover between 150 000 to 550 000 inhabitants (Table 1).

These registers are distributed throughout Europe and operate in areas with different systems of organization of medical care. This was taken into account when designing the whole project and standardization of methodology respected these differences (Fig. 4).

Until 15 February 1971 information on 4 800 patients of both sexes in the age groups of less than 65 years was collected and analyzed. The experience showed that the methodology is so far standardized that in 1971

Table 2. *EURO CVD programme. Training.*

No. of fellowships: 202
Fellowship months: 400

Courses:
- Coronary care 6
- Rehabilitation 3
- Epidemiology Special week in F & R courses

Manuals:
- Cardiovascular epidemiology (G. Rose & J. R. T. Colley, 1969)
- Intensive coronary care (M. F. Oliver & D. G. Julian, 1970)

Study on:
- Postgraduate Training in Cardiology (EURO/European Society of Cardiology)

a full-scale study could be carried out. All the record forms are pooled and centrally analyzed. This project should thus enable those involved in the studies as well as the organizers of medical care in the respective areas, to get an accurate picture of the extent of the problem in their respective community. It is possible to collect exact figures on the mortality in detailed time sequence after the onset of symptoms, information on the symptoms preceding myocardial infarction, duration of the sick leave, effects of the rehabilitation programmes on patients if applied, compared to those where no rehabilitation programmes were provided, as well as on the long-term invalidity and recurrences. Through a long-term follow-up, further data will be collected. The systems developed are used to evaluate the effects of any new organizational measure introduced with the intention to improve the medical care for patients with myocardial infarction.

A big source of information on patients with myocardial infarction in the community will thus be created. Prospective studies have been started in some places and are being planned in other areas on symptoms preceeding myocardial infarction, on effects of long-term physical training, on recurrences of myocardial infarction, and on different secondary preventive trials, as well as in the field on health economics.

It is necessary to stress that the ischaemic heart disease registers are not a pool for collecting the statistical information on the incidence of the heart attack in the community only, but their existence is only justified when they will be used as a tool for further studies, with the intention of improving the care for patients with myocardial infarction, to decrease the high death toll in the first hours after the attack and as a basis for preventing the event from the very beginning.

It is natural that these registers are a nucleus around which further activitites in the cardiovascular disease field are created. They are the first seed of Heart or CVD community control programmes. Naturally

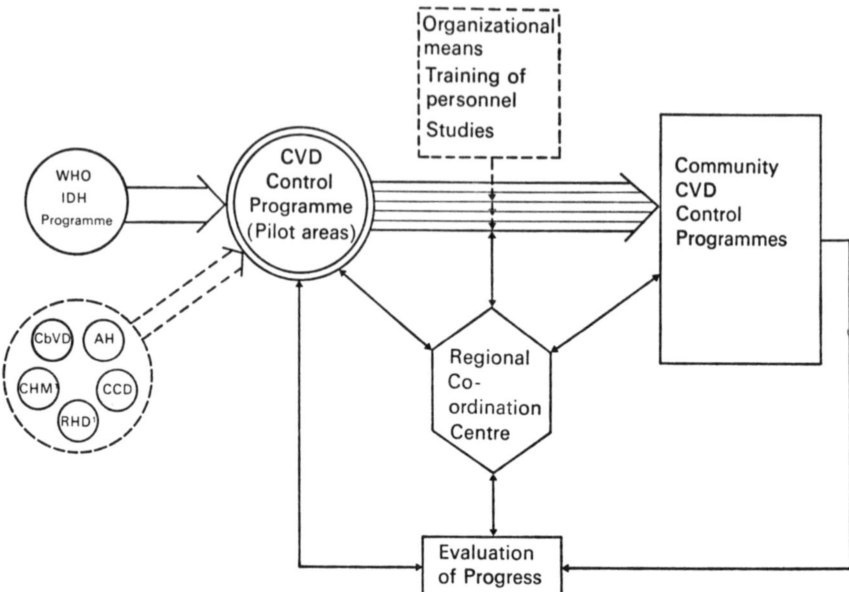

[1] to be applied according to needs of respective countries.

Fig. 5. Descriptive chart of the cardiovascular disease programme of the WHO regional office for Europe from 1973 unvards.

Abbreviations (used for this figure only): AH = arterial hypertension, CCD = chronic chest diseases leading to cor pulmonale, CHM = congenital heart malformations, CVD = cardiovascular diseases, CbVD = cerebrovascular diseases, IHD = ischaemic heart diseases, RHD = rheumatic heart diseases.

further activities on control of hypertension and stroke as well as other cardiovascular diseases have to be combined with them. In a few areas stroke registers and attempts to develop studies on community control of hypertension have already been started.

As far as the training programme is concerned, Table 2 shows the number of fellowships and fellowship months awarded in the field of cardiovascular diseases from the beginning of 1968 to 30 june 1971, by the European Office of WHO. Great importance is given to the training in epidemiological methods and in medical statistics.

The programme will continue also in the years 1973 to 1977. It is proposed to continue the activities in the field of ischaemic heart disease, to expand the programme to other cardiovascular diseases, viz. to hypertension, stroke, congenital heart malformations, chronic chest diseases leading to cor pulmonale and to rheumatic fever and rheumatic heart disease. Emphasis will be placed on prevention and education. It is envisaged that, first in pilot areas, effective cardiovascular control programmes on an experimental basis can be developed, and then all efforts should be made to simplify the methodology so that finally the wide application of CVD control programmes on a community basis could be achieved (Fig. 5).

The role of WHO is that of a co-ordinator. It can work only through the national institutes and through the national support to these institutes. The crucial task at the present time is the national co-ordination and stimulation of the activities. The public health authorities in several countries already recognized this problem and are attempting to make provision for national co-ordination of the activities, leading to control of cardiovascular diseases on a national basis.

Through this programme, an organizational structure within the frame of existing schemes of medical services in different countries is being developed and tested. It should be prepared to introduce any preventive measure in the field of CVD as soon as it is available and ensure its greatest efficiency.

The heart control programme in Finland

By Veikko Kallio

The extremely high mortality in cardiovascular diseases (CVD) in Finland is well known among the participants of this meeting. Although the hospitals are still the main means in campaign against CVD in Finland, the necessity of developing an active community oriented heart control programme has been brought into discussion. The WHO programme on CVD referred to by Dr Pisa, was thus well timed and some progress has already been made in Finland.

Many of the activities already existing or in planning phase are connected with IHD-Registers. The first Register started in Helsinki September 1969 and there are plans to continue this activity for un unlimited period of time. The second register was started in Tampere October 1970 and there are definite plans to start the register in Turku and Joensuu early next year. The population covered by these registers is about one million or about 1/4 of the whole population in Finland. The register areas give a suitable means for various kinds of experimental and methodological studies before these are being transferred to the whole country.

One of the special problems studied in Helsinki is the effectiveness of a mobile coronary care unit in reducing the mortality figures of acute myocardial infarction (AMI). Such a unit has been operating since 1st March 1971, using private funds from the Finnish Heart Association. After a pilot period of half a year the results have been encouraging and negotiations are being held between Finnish Heart Association and the City of Helsinki in order to transfer this service to be a part of Helsinki ambulance service. The multifactor preventive trial referred to by Prof. Karvonen will probably start next year.

The short-term rehabilitation studies have given interesting results. No systematic rehabilitation programme on all MI patients has,however, yet been started because there are still many unanswered problems, such as the effect of long-term physical training on the prognosis of MI patients. This problem will probably also be studied in Helsinki.

In Tampere, activities have been centered around the coronary care and especially the long-term follow-up of the resuscitated patients. Rehabilitation studies are also being made.

In Turku there are plans to study the prodromal symptoms of acute myocardial infarction and especially arrhythmias preceding the event.

The psychosocial factors and the long term effects of physical training programme in patients after myocardial infarction will also be studied.

The IHD-Register in Joensuu, North Karelia, will be used in connection of a public health experiment for the primary prevention of CHD, which will be launched early next year. This is for the first time in Finland when epidemiologists, sociologists, psychologists, and physicians are brought together to solve a nationwide health problem.

This intervention study will have two purposes. The general aim is to study how to promote health in population. The special purpose is to study the effects of an active health education and individual treatment of elevated blood pressure and other risk factors on the incidence of cardiovascular diseases. Attempts are being made to use the existing health services and voluntary members of women's home economics organization. These last mentioned active members of the team will facilitate e.g. to carry out the dietary advice which will be one part of the health educational programme of this study. The wide publicity given to the results of the seven countries' study in Finland, showing that the incidence of MI was much grater in East than in West Finland has promoted the beginning of this activity. The initiative came from the representatives of the local population and not from the side of medical profession. High expectations are connected with this health educational intervention study, which at this stage is planned to focus on methodological problems.

I am sure that one of the impacts of the IHD-Register activity in Finland is that it will again emphasize the real situation in CHD which is not demonstrable in hospital statistics. Apart from this, some useful and interesting data will be available. I have chosen some preliminary data from the Helsinki area in order to give you a few examples of the information being collected.

There are more than 1 000 new cases of AMI per year in Helsinki City in subjects less than 66 years of age. This gives an incidence of 22.7 per 10 000 people. About 4 per cent of all cases of AMI are less than 40 years of age. 53 per cent are alive after a follow up period of one year and 16 per cent only are back to their original work, according to a follow-up study of 193 cases. These figures are close to those presented from Göteborg and will be a matter for reflection for the health authorities.

Some preliminary results of the coronary ambulance service in Helsinki are now available. Among the 700 calls, there were about 350 patients with no AMI. Resuscitation was attempted on 25 patients, 14 of which were subsequently dismissed from hospital. Apart from this, there were 40–50 critically ill patients, which received antiarrhythmic on other treatment at home or during transport to hospital. The results of the short pilot study are thus in favour of establishing this service as an integral part of the general ambulance service in Helsinki.

What about the future? The possibilities to extend the notification and registration of all cases of AMI to the whole country are now being considered. This could be done using a simple notification card taking advantage of the experiences collected in the IHD-Register areas. This activity could be one of the first steps in creating a nationwide heart control programme, in the construction of which the results of the small scale studies performed in different IHD-Register areas can be used.

The heart control programme in Sweden

By Gösta Tibblin

The cardiovascular diseases dominate the picture of mortality in Sweden. An attempt to limit these diseases is to establish control programmes.

The Planning group of Preventive Cardiology of the Swedish Medical Research council started in the autumn 1970. The aim is to establish programmes for description and control of heart diseases in different parts of Sweden. The various aspects of the programmes of the participating centres are presented in Table 1. The myocardial infarction register is already established in four centres and population studies are in progress in five areas.

To give a practical example of the WHO programme the different enterprises in Göteborg will be described.

When the programme started in 1968 we discovered that after myocardial infarction post-hospital care was very heterogenous. Some patients were receiving intensive supervised physical training, but others nothing at all. This is unsatisfactory when considering that just as many patients died during the first year after an attack as during the acute hospital period. Coronary care units using the latest therapeutic techniques have increased the chance of survival for myocardial infarction patients. We will now study if these chanses can be still further improved by regular checks-ups and supervision after hospital discharge.

The follow-up of the MI patients is possible through the MI-Register. The population study of men born in 1913 has shown some important risk factors for development of myocardial infarction. In order to test the hypothesis that reducing smoking, cholesterol and high arterial blood pressure we started the Preventive trial where 10 000 men between 45 and 55

Table 1. *The heart control programme in Sweden.*

	MI-register	Stroke-register	Infarction outpatient clinic	Secondary prevention trials	Primary prevention trials	Population studies
Boden (1)	×				×	×
Falun (2)	×		×	×		
Göteborg (3)	×	×	×	×	×	×
Malmö (4)	×					×
Gävle (5)						×
Uppsala (6)					×	×

were chosen as an experimental group and another 20 000 were selected as controls receiving no treatment. The results of the trial will be evaluated by the MI- and Stroke-register.

The programmes in the six towns of Sweden offers a chance to compare costs and benefits of various forms of care provide and to find answers to many questions. How many intensive coronary care units and infarction out-patient clinics do we need? How many can we afford? What is the value of primary compared to secondary prevention? Does health education save lives?

With MI-registers working in six places there will be a possibility of comparing the distribution of different kinds of myocardial infarction with regard to patient background and clinical severity. From a pooled register it will be possible to study such homogenous sub-groups in secondary preventive trials.

A study of representative post-myocardial infarction patients aged 27–55

By Dag Elmfeldt and Lars Wilhelmsen

Myocardial infarction (MI) is an important cause of death in middle-aged and older people in Sweden (19). A great deal of the deaths occur before hospital care is reached but there is also a fairly high mortality in hospitals, which has decreased since the introduction of coronary care units (8). The mortality after hospital care has, however, not attracted as much attention as the mortality during the above-mentioned periods.

The high mortality both within and outside hospitals and the high degree of disablement in patients who have suffered a MI has called for primary and secondary preventive measures (20).

The purposes of the Post-MI clinic in Göteborg are to:

1. Validate the "primary" risk factors for MI through comparisons between representative post MI populations and random population samples.
2. Undertake follow-up studies of representative MI populations and thereby identify risk factors for death and reinfarction ("secondary risk factors").
3. Undertake secondary preventive trials in MI populations treated in a standardized and optimal manner (i.e. trials with supervised physical training, antiarrythmic drugs etc.).

An important characteristic of the Post-MI Clinic in Göteborg is that it covers the post infarction care of all patients in Göteborg in the age groups in question. It started in January 1968 and this report concerns a study in patients up to 55 years of age.

In this paper some results on mortality and postinfarction disablement are presented and furthermore some primary and secondary risk factors are presented.

Study population and methods

Göteborg is an industrial and harbour town with 450 000 inhabitants. Nearly all hospital care of MI patients is delivered at one hospital. An Ischaemic Heart Disease Register (6) has shown that virtually all diagnosed cases of MI are sent to hospital. The general autopsy rate in the hospitals and at the forensic department is very high – 92 per cent in the age-groups up to 55 years of age.

It is possible to estimate the number of previously undiagnosed, or in the I.H.D. Register unknown infarcts, due to questionnaires and ECG-recordings in an on-going cross-sectional examination which is a part of a multifactorial primary preventive study (21).

Infarct patients 55 years old or younger reported from the IHD Register, are interviewed according to a fixed protocol by the clinic doctor during hospital stay. They are informed about their disease and the benefit of a thorough follow-up after leaving hospital and are invited to the Post-MI clinic for this purpose. The attendece is 99 per cent.

Three months after the MI and then annualy the patients are seen for scheduled follow-up studies. A history is taken and physical examination is done as well as chest *X*-ray (in standing position) and an exercise ECG on bicycle ergometer. Blood samples for analysis of serum cholesterol (4), serum triglycerides (2) and for lipoprotein electrophoresis (7, 14), coagulation factors and some other variables are taken. Apart from these scheduled visits each patient is seen as often as needed from the clinical point of view. All patients are given a basic treatment aiming at optimal care of risk factors and complications. Besides this, 50 per cent of the patients have been allocated at random to supervised physical training (15).

The MI patients can be compared to the general population with the aid of results from two studies of random samples of the population; the Men Born in 1913 Study (17) and the Women Study 1968–1969 (1).

Morbidity, mortality and disablement after myocardial infarction

During the first year of the Post-MI Clinic in Göteborg, 135 cases of myocardial infarction was diagnosed in individuals 55 years old or younger. Göteborg has about 180 000 inhabitants in the ages 25–55. The youngest patient was a man aged 27. Morbidity in relation to age and sex is given in Table 1.

In Figure 1 the total number of diagnosed infarct cases during one year can be seen as well as their survival during the first 18 months. Most fatal cases died outside hospital. The figures for prehospital, hospital and post-hospital deaths were 31, 13 and 12, respectively. As expected the prognosis after an initial infarct was a bit better than after a reinfarction which is also seen in Fig. 1.

Among the 91 patients who survived the acute phase and left hospital

Table 1. Incidence of myocardial infarction (1968) in men and women (aged 25–54) in Göteborg in relation to age.

Age	Men			Women		
	Total population	Myocardial infarcts	Myocardial infarcts per 10 000	Total population	Myocardial infarcts	Myocardial infarcts per 10 000
25–29	18 327	1		16 130		
30–34	13 723			12 340		
35–39	12 985	3	2	12 390	1	1
40–44	14 256	19	13	14 040	1	1
45–49	16 369	31	19	16 594	3	2
50–54	14 467	61	42	15 370	4	3
25–54	90 127	115		86 864	9	

the one year mortality for initial infarction was 10 per cent, for reinfarction 20 per cent.

The survival rate and the state of working capacity at the end of the first year after the infarct is illustrated in Figure 2. By the end of the year 40 per cent were dead, 15 per cent were drawing sickness benefit, 10 per cent needed a lighter work and just some 35 per cent were back in the same work as before the infarct.

Besides morbidity and mortality data it is of great interest to study disablement after a MI. In Figure 3 the prevalence of angina pectoris according to a standardized questionnaire before and 3 and 12 months after the

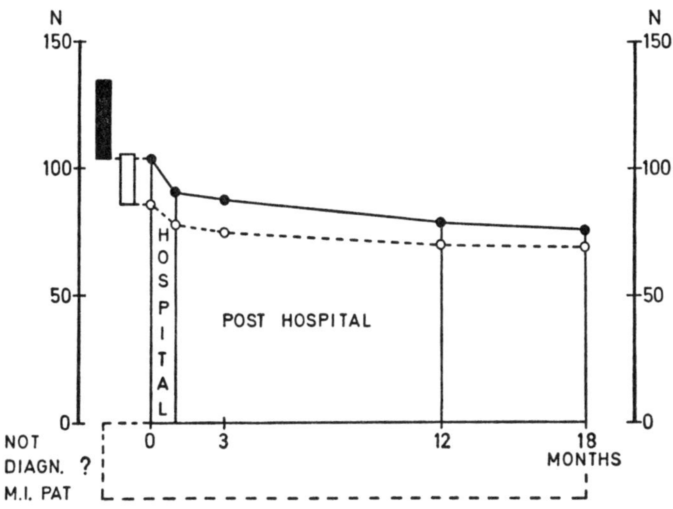

Fig. 1. Survival after myocardial infarction among men and women 55 years old or younger living in Göteborg. All cases during one year (1968). The bars to the left indicate fatal cases before hospital contact was established.
Filled bar all cases. Open bar initial infarcts. The Post-MI Clinic, Göteborg.

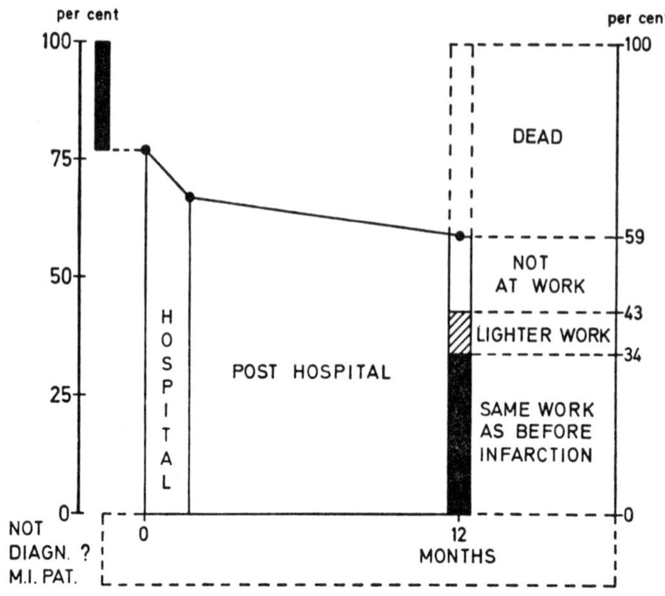

Fig. 2. Survival and return to work in per cent of all cases of myocardial infarction in men and women 55 years old or younger during one year (1968) in Göteborg. One year follow up. Total number 135. The bar to the left indicates fatal cases before hospital contact was established. The Post-MI Clinic, Göteborg.

infarct is presented. Almost 50 per cent of patients with an initial infarct had angina. The figure for those with reinfarction was 70 per cent. Dyspnea was also quite common as shown in Figure 4. At the end of the first year about 35 per cent had this symptom.

Primary risk factors in the post infarct period

The mean serum cholesterol level in the total male patient group (age 27–55, mean 49) three months after the infarct was found to be elevated ($p < 0.01$) when compared to the level of a random population sample of men aged 55. Related to age groups the difference was significant only for patients aged 40 or younger ($p < 0.05$). These young patients also showed an elevated mean serum cholesterol level in comparison with the older patients' ($p < 0.05$), Figure 5.

Compared to the control group of 55 years old men serum triglycerides were significantly higher both for the total patient group ($p < 0.01$) and for the breakdown in age-groups ($p < 0.05$) with the exception of the group of men aged 41–45, Figure 6.

The distribution of serum lipoprotein types in the random sample and

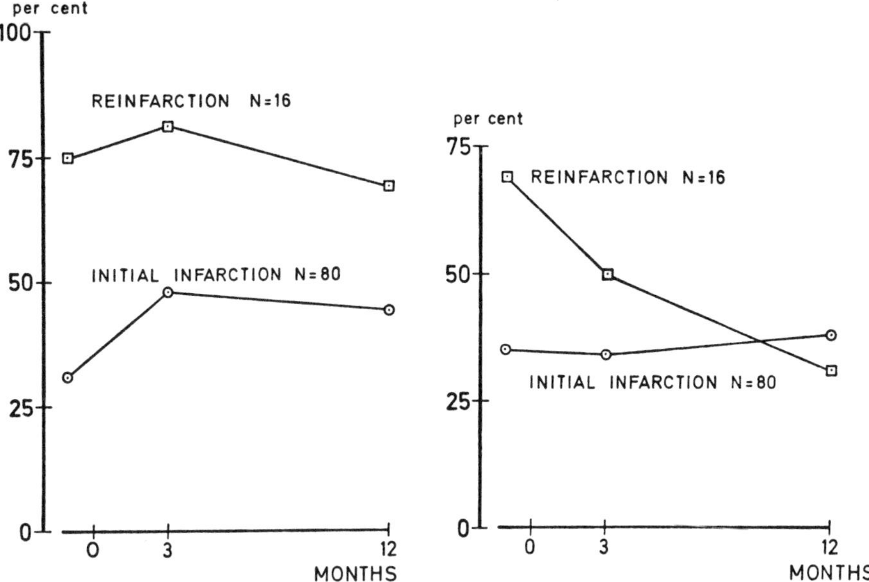

Fig. 3. Angina pectoris according to a standardized questionnaire before and 3 months and 12 months after myocardial infarction. Per cent of patients with initial infarct and with reinfact. Men and women 55 years old or younger. The Post-MI Clinic, Göteborg.

Fig. 4. Dyspnea according to a standardized questionnaire before and 3 months and 12 months after myocardial infarction. Per cent of patients with initial infarct and with reinfarct. Men and women 55 years old or younger. The Post-MI Clinic, Göteborg.

in the patients (related to age) three months after their MI is presented in Figure 7. Abnormal types were much more common among patients than among controls. This was most obvious in the youngest age group where a very high proportion of type II A and II B, e.g. II with pre-beta-lipoproteins was found.

Hypertension, diabetes, smoking and physical inactivity were much more prevalent in this population of patients with MI than in the general population (22).

Risk factors for death during the post hospital stage after a myocardial infarction (secondary risk factors)

One factor in the history concerning cardiovascular symptoms *before* the infarct was found to discriminate between a group with high and another group with low one-year-mortality after having left hospital. That symptom was dyspnea defined as breathlessness walking uphill. Ten out of 88, e.g. 12 per cent, with this symptom were dead at the end of the first year

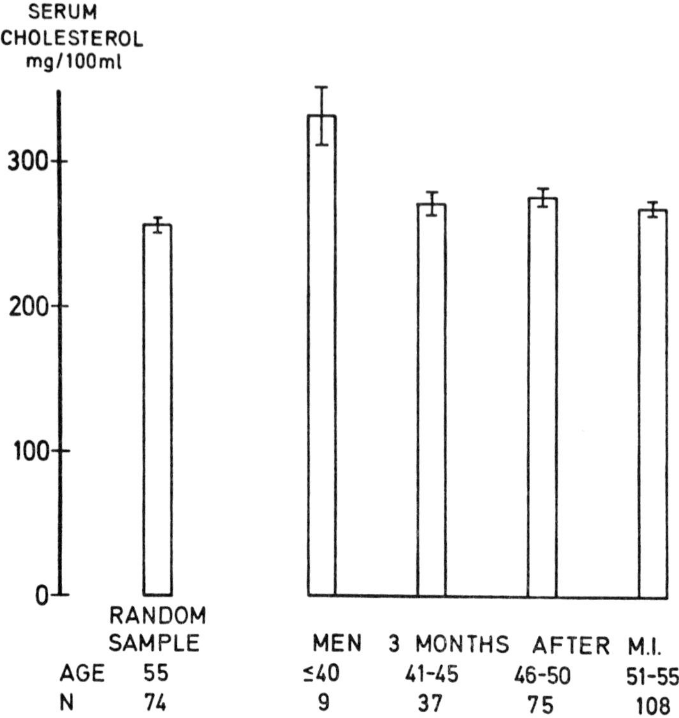

Fig. 5. Serum cholesterol (mean ± S.E.M.) in relation to age in men (aged 27–55, mean 49) 3 months after their myocardial infarction and in a random sample of 55 years old men. The Post-MI clinic, Göteborg.

compared to 5 out of 126 or 4 per cent of those without dyspnea before the MI, Figure 8. This difference was not due to the higher prevalence of dyspnea in cases with reinfarction, having a higher one-year mortality.

Left heart failure and heart enlargement during the acute stage were associated with bad risk as shown in Figure 9. Left heart failure was defined as physically and/or roentgenologically diagnosed pulmonary congestion. Heart enlargement was defined as a heart volume on *X*-ray over the mean value for the patients, e.g. 440 ml/m^2 body surface area.

Other variables indicating extended myocardial damage (i.e. high maximum serum transaminases, high maximum body temperature) were also identified as secondary risk factors.

Atrial fibrillation and/or atrial flutter as well as ventricular tachycardia occurring during hospital care were also risk factors for death during the first year after the MI.

None of the primary risk factors (smoking, high blood lipids, hypertension, low physical activity) were of prognostic significance during the first year following the infarct.

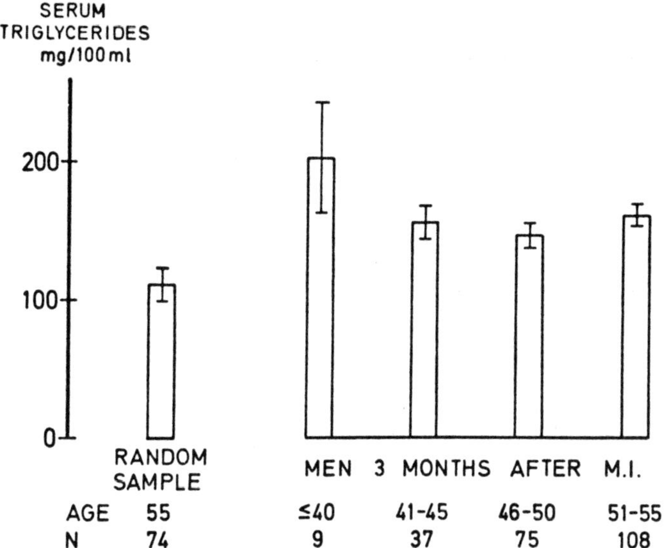

Fig. 6. Serum triglycerides (mean ± S.E.M.) in relation to age in men (age 27–55, mean 49) 3 months after their myocardial infarction and in a random sample of 55 years old men. The Post-MI Clinic, Göteborg.

Discussion

The findings of high serum cholesterol in post infarct patients is in agreement with several studies showing cholesterol as a primary risk factor for MI (5, 9, 11, 16, 23). After an infarct a decrease of the serum cholesterol level is known to follow (18).

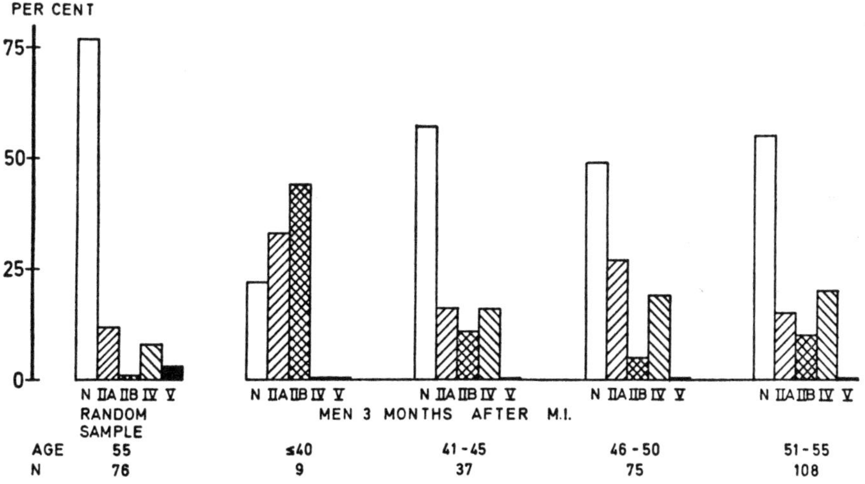

Fig. 7. Serum lipoprotein types in relation to age in men (age 27–55, mean 49) 3 months after their myocardial infarction and in a random sample of 55 years old men. The Post-MI Clinic, Göteborg.

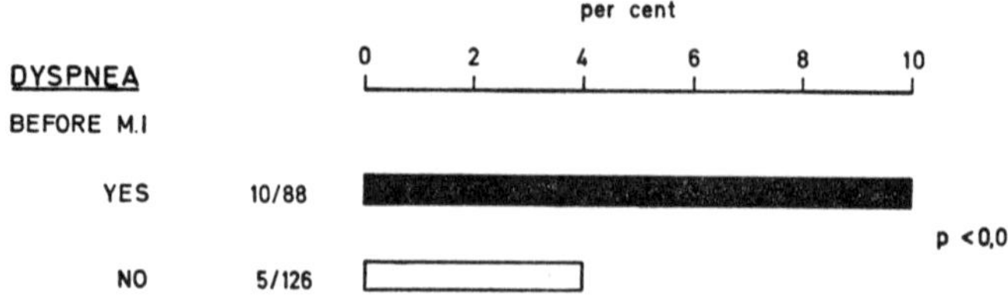

Fig. 8. One year mortality after being sent home from hospital after myocardial infarction. Mortality related to dyspnea, defined as breathlessness walking uphill, before the infarct. Men and women 55 years old or younger. The Post-MI Clinic, Göteborg.

So, if anything, the differences found by us are minimum, as in some cases the original serum level might not have been reached 3 months after the MI. Since the cholesterol level increases with increasing age (3), the finding of very high cholesterol in the youngest patients is a strong indication of this virtually being an important deviation from normal in young infarct patients. In older age MI seems to occur with less disturbed cholesterol values.

Serum triglycerides are known to increase after an infarct (18). They show the highest levels in the normal population in age 40–50 (3). These facts may explain part of, but hardly all, the difference found between patients and controls in this study. In prospective population studies this variable has also been found to be a risk factor for MI (23).

In this investigation, it has been possible to study only those patients who survived their MI and there is some uncertainty as to the risk factors in those who died outside hospital. The Framingham Study has, however, shown that these subjects are more heavily afflicted with high blood lipids than those who survive (10).

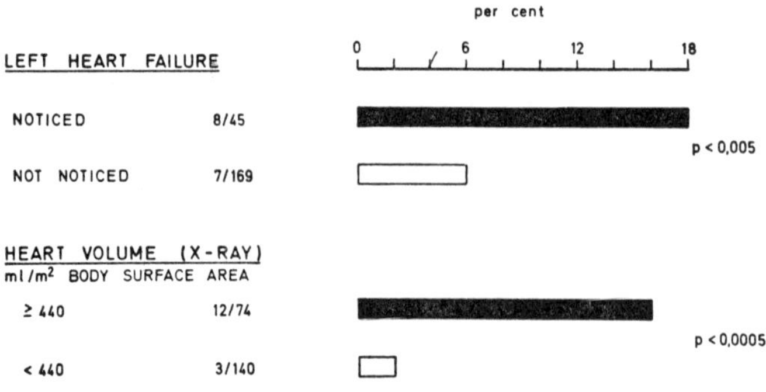

Fig. 9. One year mortality after being sent home from hospital after myocardial infarction. Mortality related to left heart failure and to heart enlargement during the acute stage. Men and women 55 years old or younger. The Post-MI Clinic, Göteborg.

The very high mortality outside hospital calls for prevention and it is obvious that still higher technical standard and more coronary care units can not radically reduce total mortality. Preventive measures must be of primary type in order to decrease the total amount of initial infarcts and of secondary type aiming to decrease the post hospital deaths and disablement. More knowledge about premonitory symptoms and treatment of early arrythmias and education of persons at risk could possibly contribute in decreasing the prehospital deaths.

It is of interest that the primary risk factors did not work as risk factors for death during the first year of follow-up. The secondary risk factors were closely related to the extent of the myocardial damage, e.g. enlargement of the heart, left heart failure, high temperature and high serum transaminases etc. during the acute phase. Such factors have been shown in other studies to be correlated to bad prognosis during the acute stage too (13). Primary risk factors may be of importance as risk factors for death during a longer follow up period (12).

In patients who entered the study because of a reinfarction there was a considerable decrease of dyspnea during the follow-up. This illustrates the need for adequate post coronary care since the vanishing of this symptom was correlated to digitalization. The reason why dyspnea before MI is a risk factor for later death is not known. Earlier MI can be excluded as had already been pointed out. Lack of physical activity which has been claimed to be of prognostic importance can probably also be excluded as the explanation since low physical activity before the infarct was not found to be a secondary risk factor.

Atrial fibrillation and flutter and ventricular tachycardia were secondary risk factors but not ventricular extrasystolies during the hospital period. This does not, however, exclude the possibility that these are of prognostic significance as so called malignant extrasystolies were rarely recorded.

Summary

All myocardial infarct cases during one year in Göteborg were registered and all nonfatal cases were followed for at least one year. The incidence of myocardial infarction in people aged 55 or younger was found to be 70/100 000/year. About 10 per cent were women. The one year mortality was 40 per cent and the amount of disablement was conciderable. High serum cholesterol level and high serum triglycerides as well as abnormal lipoprotein types were shown to be overrepresented three months after the infarct in male patients (especially in the youngest age-group), when compared to a representative population sample. The same stands for other well known primary risk factors as smoking, hypertension, diabetes and physical inactivity. Risk factors for death during the first post coronary year were found among factors known to correlate with extended myocardial damage. None of the so called primary risk factors worked as secondary risk factors during the first post hospital year.

Acknowledgements

This study has been supported by grants from the Swedish Medical Research Council (B 71 – 61 P – 3211 – 01) and the Swedish National Association against Heart and Chest Diseases. Our thanks are due to Anders Gustavsson, M.D. who made the lipid analysis and the lipoprotein typing.

References

1. Bengtsson, C.: The Woman Study 1968–1969. *Pehr Dubb J.*, III (4) 14, 1969.
2. Carlsson, L. A.: Determination of serum glycerides. *Acta Soc. Med. Upsalien. 64:* 208, 1959.
3. Carlsson, L. A. & Lindstedt, S.: The Stockholm Prospective Study I. The initial value for plasma lipids. *Acta Med. Scand.,* Suppl. 493, 1969.
4. Cramér, K. & Isaksson, B.: An evaluation of the Theorell method for the determination of total serum cholesterol. *Scand. J. Clin. Lab. Invest. 11:* 213, 1959.
5. Epstein, F. H.: The epidemiology of coronary heart disease. *J. Chron. Dis. 18:* 735, 1965.
6. Fodor, J.: The Ischaemic Heart Disease Register in Göteborg–a Pilot study. *Pehr Dubb J.* III (4) 26, 1969.
7. Fredrickson, D. S.: A system for pheno-typing hyperlipoproteinemia. *Circulation 31:* 321, 1965.
8. Hofvendahl, S.: Influence of treatment in a coronary care unite on prognosis in acute myocardial infarction. *Acta Med. Scand.,* Suppl. 519, 1971.
9. Kannel, W. B.: Results of the epidemiologic investigation of ischaemie heart disease: illustrated by the Framingham Study. In *Ischaemic heart disease* (ed.) J. H. de Haas, H. C. Hemker & H. A. Snellen. Leiden University Press, 1970.
10. Kannel, W. B., Castelli, W. P. & McNamara, P. M.: The coronary profile– 12-year follow up in the Framingham Study. *J. Occup. Med., 9:* 611, 1967.
11. Keys, A. (Ed.): Coronary heart disease in seven countries. *Circulation 41:* Suppl. 1, 1970.
12. Leren, P.: The Oslo diet–heart study. Eleven year report. *Circulation 42*: 935, 1970.
13. Norris, R. M., Brandt, P. W. T. & Canghey, D. E.: A new coronary prognostic index. *Lancet I3* 274, 1969.
14. Rapp, W. & Kahlke, W.: Lipoprotein–electrophorese in agarose gel. *Clin. Chem. Acta. 19:* 493, 1968.
15. Sanne, H., Grimby, G. & Wilhelmsson, L.: Physical training during convalescense after a myocardial infarction. In *Coronary heart disease and physical fitness* (ed.) O. Andrée-Larsen, & R. O. Malmborg, Munksgaard, Copenhagen, 1971.

16. Stamler, J.: Prevention by change of diet and mode of life. In *Iscaemic heart disease* (ed.) J. H. de Haas, H. C. Hemker, & H. A. Snellen, Leiden University Press, 1970.
17. Tibblin, G.: High blood pressure in men aged 50–A population study of men born in 1913. *Acta Med. Scand.,* Suppl. 470, 1967.
18. Tibblin, G. & Cramér, K.: Serum lipids during the cause of an acute myocardial infarction and one year afterwards. *Acta Med. Scand. 174:* 451, 1965.
19. Vedin, A. J., Wilhelmsson, C.-E., Bolander, A.-M. & Werkö, L. Mortality trends in Sweden 1951–1968 with special reference to cardiovascular causes of death. *Acta Med. Scand.,* Suppl. 515, 1971.
20. Werkö, L.: Can we prevent heart disease? *Ann. Int. Med. 74:* 278, 1971.
21. Wilhelmsen, L., Tibblin, G. & Werkö, L.: *Prevent. Med 1:* 153, 1972.
22. Wilhelmsen, L.: The Myocardial Infarction Clinic in Göteborg–organization and preliminary results. *Pehr Dubb. J.,* (III) 4, 43, 1969.
23. Wilhelmsen, L. & Tibblin, G.: Physical inactivity and risk of myocardial infarction–The Men Born in 1913 Study. In *Coronary heart disease and physical fitness* (ed.) O. Andrée-Larsen & R. O. Malmborg, Munksgaard, Copenhagen, 1971.

Myocardial infarction in young women

By Calle Bengtsson

As myocardial infarction is rare in young women—much more rare than in young men—the clinical features of myocardial infarction in women have not been much studied, nor do we know much about what we call "risk factors" for myocardial infarction in women. Clinical materials of young women with myocardial infarction have been small. This is to be said about our material in Göteborg, too, but there are three things of special interest with this material which makes it quite unique. Firstly it comprises the total number of women with clinical myocardial infarction in a defined area, secondly the population of the same defined are has been studied by means of two population studies, the Men born in 1913 Study (3) and the Study of Women 1968–1969 (1) making a comparison between subjects with myocardial infarction and the total population in the same area and the same ages possible. Thirdly, as the men in the same area have been studied in the same way comparisons between men and women may be made.

The purpose with this paper is to give some characteristics of the women with myocardial infarction and compare them with those from the population study in the same ages in order to see, whether there are any differences between the women with myocardial infarction and those of the population. From the population study, those in the age strata 50 and 54 were chosen, altogether 578 women, who had almost exactly the same mean age as the women with myocardial infarction.

Material

All persons in Göteborg, born in 1913 or later, surviving an acute attack of myocardial infarction are registered in a special register since the 1st of January 1968 (2). The present material comprises the 45 women with myocardial infarction during the first three years, thus during 1968, 1969 and 1970. As they were born in 1913 or later, none of them was more than 57 years of age. The sex ratio man to woman was about 7 to 1. The annual incidence rate increased in the women from about 3 per 100 000 in the ages 35–39 to 40 per 100 000 in the ages 50–54, including "sudden death" from 5 to 60 respectively.

Table 1. *History of previous myocardial infarction and some symptoms in women with myocardial infarction (MI) as compared to women in the population.*

History of	Women with MI (per cent)	Population study (per cent)	χ^2-test
Chest pain	68.9	6.4	$p<0.001$
Chest pain confirming the diagnosis of angina pectoris	44.4	3.3	$p<0.001$
Myocardial infarction	11.1	—	$p<0.001$
Breathlessness	60.0	21.2	$p<0.001$
Intermittent claudication	9.3	0.9	$p<0.001$

Results

Prevalence of previous myocardial infarction and symptoms

As seen from Table 1 more than 10 per cent of the women with myocardial infarction had a history of previous myocardial infarction and almost half of them had a history of angina pectoris. History of breathlessness and intermittent claudication was also much more common in the myocardial infarction women as compared to the women in the population study. All these differences were highly significant and are similar to those found in the male series.

Social data

Table 2 shows some social data. No differences of importance were found between the women with myocardial infarction and those in the population study.

Risk factors

There are several well-established risk factors for myocardial infarction in men. We know less about these in women. In Table 3 the prevalence of some risk factors for myocardial infarction are given.

Table 2. *Social data in women with myocardial infarction (MI).*

Social data	Women with MI (per cent)	Population study (per cent)	χ^2-test
Born in the Göteborg area	56.0	52.4	$p>0.10$
Married	80.4	76.3	$p>0.10$
Have children	78.0	79.3	$p>0.10$
Wage-earning outside home	52.5	64.2	$p>0.10$

Table 3. *Prevalence of probable risk factors in women with myocardial infarction as compared to women in the population.*

Prevalence of "risk factors"	Women with MI (per cent)	Population study (per cent)	χ^2-test
Hypertension	44.4	12.3	$p<0.001$
Diabetes	13.3	0.9	$p<0.001$
Smoking	79.4	37.3	$p<0.001$
"Severe stress"	47.2	19.9	$p<0.001$

Hypertension. Hypertension was much more common in the myocardial infarction women, thus almost half of them had a history of hypertension as compared to somewhat more than 10 per cent in the women from the population study of corresponding age.

Diabetes mellitus. Thirteen per cent of the women with myocardial infarction had history of diabetes mellitus as compared to 0.9 per cent in the population.

Smoking. Eighty per cent of the women with myocardial infarction were smokers as compared to less than 40 per cent in the population.

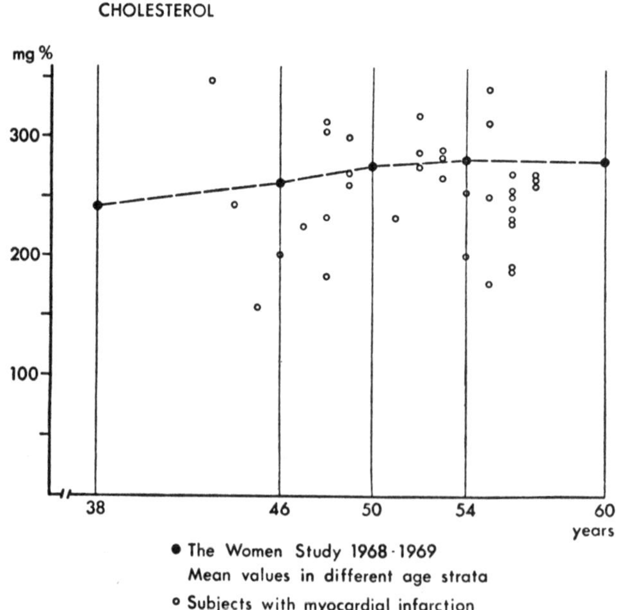

Fig. 1. Serum cholesterol in women with myocardial infarction 3 months after the infection as compared to mean values of women in different age strata in the population.

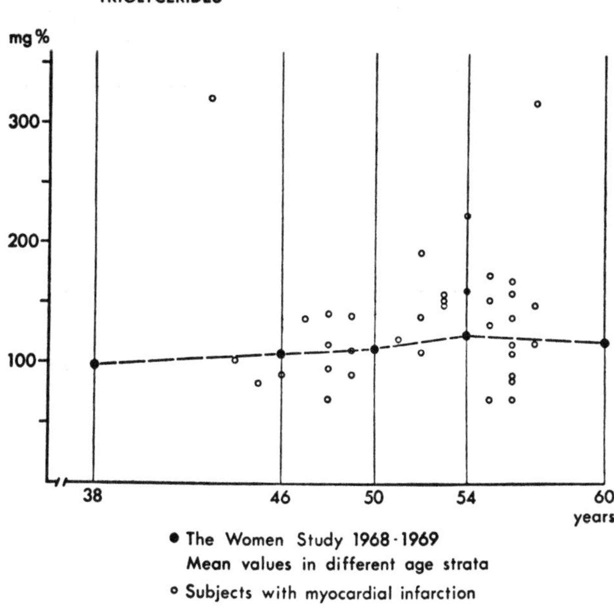

Fig. 2. Serum triglycerides in women with myocardial infarction 3 months after the infarction as compared to mean values of women in different age strata in the population.

Stress. "Severe stress" defined as several periods of feeling of stress during a month or longer including anxiety, nervousness, fear and sleeplessness in connection with conflicts during the last 5 years, was reported in almost half of the women with myocardial infarction against 20 per cent in the population. We have to be very cautious when discussing stress, as these women with myocardial infarction were interviewed after their infarction, which may have influenced their way of answering.

Blood lipids. Cholesterol and triglycerides were studied 3 months after the infarction. In Fig. 1 and 2 the individual values of the myocardial infarc-

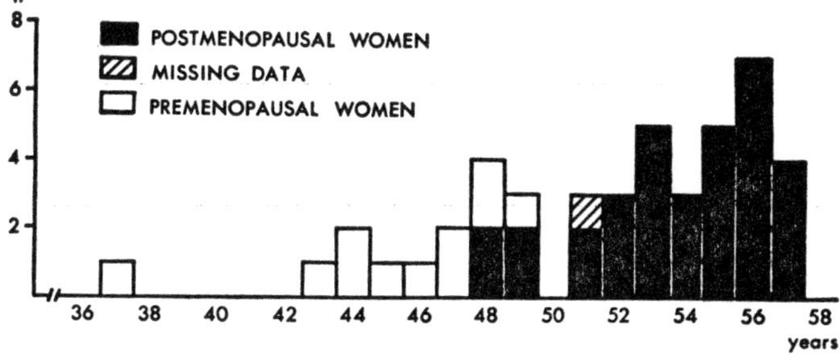

Fig. 3. Age and menopausal stage in women with myocardial infarction.

Table 4. *Number of postmenopausal women (per cent) at the age of 40, 45 and 50 respectively in women with myocardial infarction (MI) as compared to women in the population.*

	Women with MI (per cent)	Population study (per cent)	χ^2-test
Menopause at the age of 40	8.9	4.0	$p>0.10$
Menopause at the age of 45	22.7	11.6	$p<0.05$
Menopause at the age of 50	74.3	48.4	$p<0.01$

tion women are given in relation to age. The dotted lines connect the mean values for cholesterol and triglycerides respectively in the different age strata as found in the population study. We did not find any higher cholesterol values for infarction women than in women in the population as seen from Figure 1. As seen from Figure 2 the same was found for triglycerides: just the same number of women above as below the line for the means of the population.

Early menopausal age. As seen from Figure 3 myocardial infarction may occur both in premenopausal and postmenopausal women. At least 11 women of 45 were thus still menstruating at the time when they had their myocardial infarction. However, the women with myocardial infarction reached the menopausal age somewhat earlier than the women in the population as seen from Table 4. The differences were statistically significant at the age of 50 and 54.

Oral contraceptive pills. The rôle of oral contraceptive pills as risk factor for myocardial infarction in young women has recently been much debated. In this material none of the 42 surviving women who have been interviewedhad ever used pills. Table 5 shows that oral contraceptive pills were in quite common use in Göteborg at this time.

Table 5. *Use of oral contraceptive pills in Göteborg as found from the population study.*

Age	Used or had used pills (per cent)	Still on pills (per cent)
38	24.4	16.1
46	7.5	1.6
50	2.6	—
54	1.8	—
60	—	—

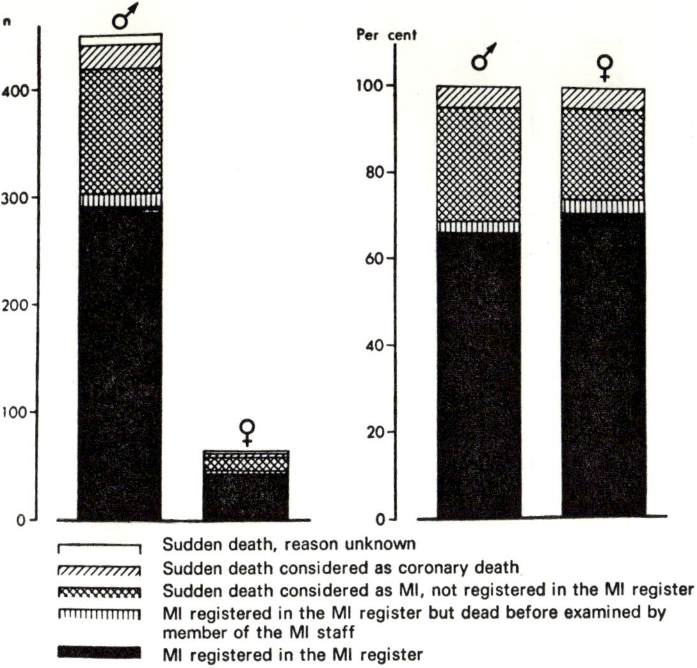

Fig. 4. Subjects born in 1913 or later living in Göteborg with myocardial infarction or unexpected "sudden death" during the years 1968–1970.

Mortality

The myocardial infarction register includes women coming to the hospital as survivors. Figure 4 also includes those dying suddenly outside hospital and comparison is made between men and women. Subjects with "sudden death" considered as myocardial infarction included those who were found to have a fresh myocardial infarction area at autopsy or history of severe chest pain in connection with death. Subjects with "sudden death" considered as coronary death included those who at autopsy were found to have prominent atheromatosis of the coronary arteries but no verified history of severe chest pain in connection with death and no fresh myocardial infarction area at autopsy. As seen from Figure 4 men predominated both by number and proportion, although the difference in per cent was not statistically significant. Figure 5 also includes those dead during a follow-up period of 1/2–3 1/2 years, mean observation time 2 years. Two women died during this follow-up period. This means that life expectancy is rather good in women surviving an acute attack of myocardial infarction and seems to be better than in men, though this difference was not statistically significant.

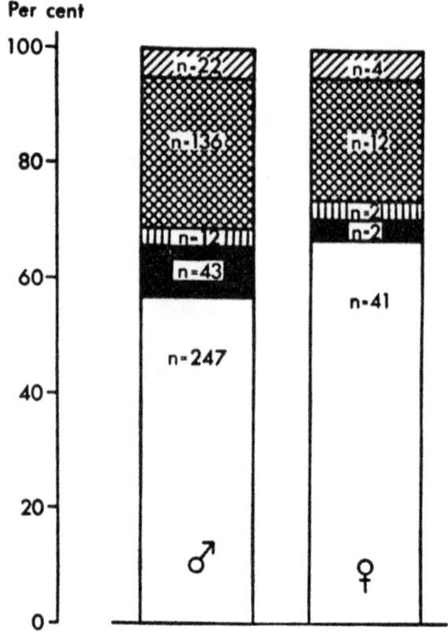

Fig. 5. Subjects born in 1913 or later living in Göteborg with definite or probable myocardial infarction during the years 1968–1970.

Discussion

Hypertension, diabetes mellitus, smoking and "severe stress" were much more common in women with myocardial infarction than in the population of corresponding age and seemed to be definite risk factors for myocardial infarction also in women. It was somewhat surprising to find that blood lipids were not higher in the women with myocardial infarction than in the population.

A very interesting question is why myocardial infarction is so much more rare in women than in men. Can it be explained by sex differences in risk factors? When comparing data from the two population studies performed in Göteborg, the Men born in 1913 Study and the Study of Women 1968–1969, we found that blood pressure was almost the same in men and women, that there were no differences of importance in cholesterol or triglycerides, and that the prevalence of diabetes mellitus was the same. However, the hematocrit was higher in the men than in the women and smoking was more common in men than in women. Probably the feeling of stress was also more common in men than women.

Summary

Forty-five women surviving an acute attack of myocardial infarction were compared with a randomized sample of women from the population in the corresponding age. History of previous myocardial infarction, angina pectoris, breathlessness and intermittent claudication was much more common in the women with myocardial infarction. No differences were found concerning social data. Hypertension, diabetes mellitus, smoking and "severe stress" were much more common in women with myocardial infarction than in the population. Cholesterol and triglycerides 3 months after myocardial infarction did not differ from those found in the population. Women with myocardial infarction reached the menopausal age somewhat earlier than those in the population but it was to be noticed that at least 11 of 45 women were still menstruating at the time when they had their infarction. None of the women had ever used oral contraceptive pills.

References

1. Bengtsson, C.: The Woman Study 1968–1969. Presentation of the investigation, and some preliminary results from the study of coronary arthery disease, blood lipids, arterial blood pressure, and smoking habits. *Pehr Dubb. J. 4:* 14–19, 1969.
2. Fodor, J.: The ischaemic hart disease register in Göteborg. A pilot study 1.11.68–31.1.69. *Pehr Dubb J. 4:* 26–33, 1969.
3. Tibblin, G.: High blood pressure in men aged 50 a population study in men born in 1913. *Acta Med. Scand.,* Suppl. 470, 1967.

The Stroke Register in Göteborg

By Per Harmsen, Göran Berglund, Ove Larsson,
Sverre Sörenson and Gösta Tibblin

Stroke cases constitutes an important part of the group of cardiovascular diseases. In view of this and in view of the fact that epidemiologic knowledge of cerebrovascular diseases is insufficient, especially when compared with the knowledge obtained over the past 10–15 years from epidemiologic studies of ischemic heart diseases, the Heart Control Programme of Gothenburg was in January 1970 extended to include a stroke register. This has the following aims:

1. to collect information for a descriptive epidemiologic analysis – to further describe natural history of stroke,
2. to describe and to evaluate diagnostic and therapeutic measures undertaken both in the acute and in the chronic phase of stroke,
3. possibly to give base-line data for a cost-benefit analysis.

I shall shortly outline the method used and the type of results obtainable referring to the first period, 1st January until 30th June 1970.

The outline of registration has been that after notification of "suspected stroke" the patient was examined and all cases of stroke occurring in persons living in the city of Gothenburg born 1904 or later have been registered. Stroke has here been defined as rapidly developed clinical signs of focal (or global) disturbance of cerebral function of presumed vascular origin and of more than a few minutes duration. From each such case the following information was sought: name, address, date of birth, date and time of admission or "contact" with medical services, length of hospitalization, diagnosis at discharge. If dead, the date and time of death, and the results of autopsy. Further: sex, marital state, physical activity at work, smoking habits, habits of alcohol consumption, heredity for cardiac and cerebrovascular diseases. Previous medical history, especially cardiovascular diseases including hypertension and diabetes, and other (non-vascular) diseases. Further, clinical findings at first medical examination, laboratory results of blood haemoglobin, creatinine and lipids, and finally results from lumbar puncture, *X*-ray of skull, echo and isotope-encephalography and angiography, had these been performed.

The total number of cases registered between 1st January – 30th June 1970 was 102. This gives an incidence of 52 per 100 000 population and year for the age group of 65 years and younger.

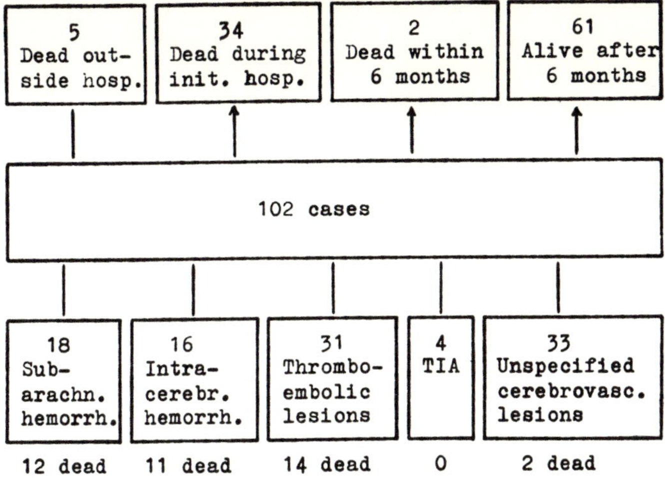

Fig. 1. Diagnosis and follow-up results.

A presentation of the material is given in Figure 1: The lower boxes give the distribution in diagnostic groups based on clinical and/or autopsy findings. The initial mortality (during the initial hospital stay) for each diagnostic group is also given in the figure.

The upper boxes give an assay of the prognosis for all cases. The five cases dead outside hospital consisted of two men and three women all above 53 years of age, four had subarachnoid hemorrhage and one intracerebral hemorrhage shown at autopsy. About one third of the patients died during the initial hospital stay.

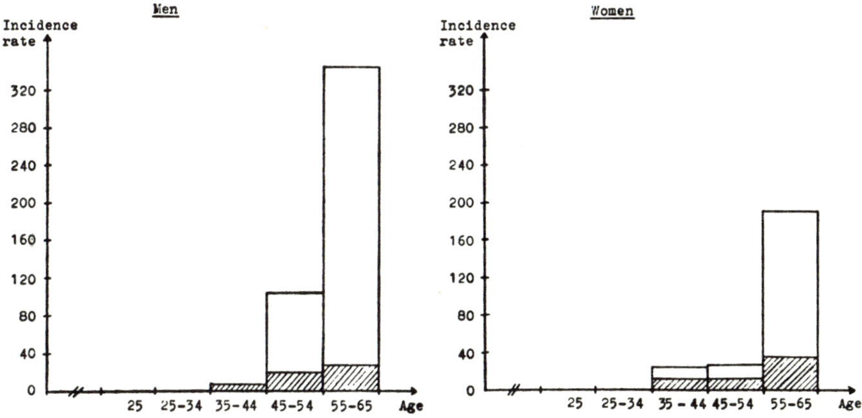

Fig. 2. Distribution of SAH (▨) and "other stroke cases" (□) by sex and age groups.

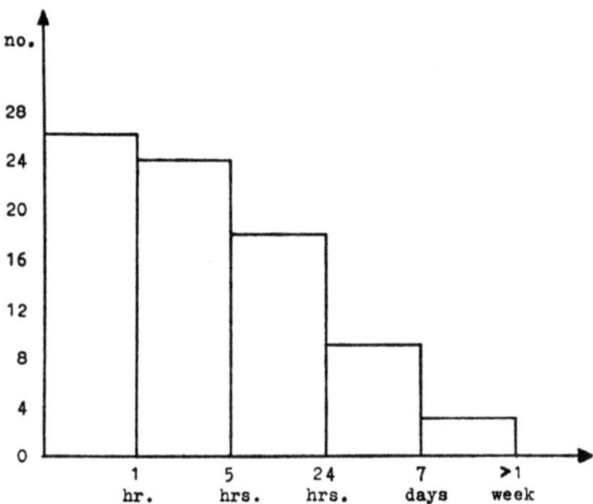

Fig. 3. Time from onset of symptoms until contact with medical services. N=80.

The distribution for males and females by age appears in Figure 2 calculated as incidence (number per 100 000 population and year for each age group and sex respectively). The overall numbers increase with age, but it also appears that there is a preponderance of male stroke cases over female. This seems to be so particularly in the younger age group (45)54) for stroke cases other than subarachnoid hemorrhage (SAH). The total male/female ratio is nearly 2: 1, (65 male and 37 female cases).

Figure 3 illustrates the time from onset of symptoms until contact with medical services in cases where this information was obtained. The great majority of patients came under medical care within the first 24 hours, only vere few appeared after one week.

In Table 1 the patients are grouped according to level of consciousness on admission and to the relation to diagnosis and initial prognosis. Around 60 % of the patients were fully awake on arrival to hospital. The distribution between diagnostic groups does not show any special trends. There

Table 1. *Level of consciousness at admission and initial mortality.*

		Cerebrovasc. diagnosis		Discharged	
	No.	SAH	Other strokes	Alive	Dead
Awake	56	4	52	49	7
Somnolent	20	6	14	11	9
Semicoma	2	0	2	0	2
Coma	15	4	11	3	12
Missing data	4	0	4	0	4
Total no. hosp. cases	97				

Table 2. *Diagnostic measures performed in 97 stroke cases served at hospital (information not retrievable in 4 cases).*

	Performed	Not performed
Lumbar puncture	47	46
X-ray of scull	45	48
Echo-encephalography	58	35
Isotope-encephalography	17	76
Cerebral angiography	33	60

Table 3. *Relation of performed lumbar puncture and diagnostic group (hospital served cases).*

	Lumb. pct. performed	Lumb. pct. not performed
Subarachnoid hemorrhage	13	1
Intracerebral hemorrhage	9	6
Thrombo-embolic lesion	15	13
TIA only	2	2
Unspecified cerebrovasc. lesion	8	24
Total no.	47	46

was as expected a pronounced increase in mortality in the patients admitted comatose.

Some diagnostic measures are listed in Table 2 with the number of cases in which they had been performed. Sometimes they might be characterized as "special examinations" and would not have been carried out unless clinical indications were present. To some extent this table also reflects the extent of diagnostic activity.

The diagnostic group to which the stroke case was referred (and here autopsy diagnoses are also included) to a large extent depended upon whether cerebrospinal fluid was examined or not (Table 3). Information on this item was lacking in 4 cases.

Table 4. *Co-existent and previous diseases in stroke cases.*

	Men (65)		"Men born 1913"	Women (37)		"Women study"
	No.	%	%	No.	%	%
Heart disease	27	43	6.4	10	29	5.3
Hypertension	30	48	7.8	16	47	10.9
Diabetes	8	13	0.8	3	9	1
Previous cerebro-vascular disease	22	35	0.3	8	23	—

Table 5. *Blood pressure at first medical examination of hospital served cases and initial mortality, in 5 cases initial BP was not retrievable.*

	No.	Discharged	
		Alive	Dead
⩾200 systolic and/or ⩾120 diast.	30	18	12
160–199 systolic and 95–119 diast.	33	23	10
<160 systolic and/or <95 diast.	29	22	7
BP unknown	5	0	5
Total no.	97		

The presence of other cardiovascular diseases in the patients with stroke and the frequency of previous cerebrovascular disease in shown in Table 4. The values are listed together with prevalence values from the two population studies from Göteborg: "Men born 1913" (at follow-up examination in 1967) and the "Women study", the age groups of which are both 54 years. As the mean ages for the male stroke patients was 57 years and for the female patients 58 years this permits a fairly adequate comparison. The stroke patients had a markedly increased frequency of heart diseases (the vast majority being ischemic), hypertension and diabetes. This difference is more pronounced in the male patients, being 5–10 times the prevalence in the population. Of the 19 male patients with previous cerebrovascular disease 10 had had this in the form of transient ischemic attacks (TIA) only. In the female patients this was the case with one only. Other non-vascular diseases were also represented with a high frequency in the stroke patients (around 50 %).

High blood pressure measured on admission is usually not recognized as any reliable sign of hypertensive disease. A blood pressure above 160

Table 6. *Electrocardiogram and cerebrovascular diagnosis of 97 hospital served cases.*

	Total no.	Cerebrovascular diagnosis				
		SAH	Intra-cerebral hemorrh.	Trombo-embolic lesion	TIA only	Unspecified cerebrovasc. lesion
Ecg normal	38	4	4	12	0	18
Ecg: signs of left ventr. dominance and/or "ischemia"	35	5	10	10	1	9
Ecg: fibrillation or flutter	7	0	0	4	1	2
Ecg not done	12	4	1	3	2	2
Ecg unknown	5	1	0	2	0	2
Total no.	97					

systolic and/or 95 diastolic gave in this series a poor prognosis (Table 5). A further analysis of these data showed that a high proportion (63 %) of those with raised blood pressure had in fact hypertensive disease. The vast majority of intracerebral hemorrhages were found in this group.

Electrocardiography had been performed in 82 % of cases (information was missing in five cases). When signs of fibrillation or flutter had been found, the diagnosis turned out to fall within the groups thrombo-embolic lesions, transient ischemic attacks or unspecified lesions (Table 6).

Finally I would mention that we are aware of a number of factors which are as yet not studied and that the study of these is necessary in order to substantiate even the trends that were here mentioned as results.

Preventive effect of physical training after a myocardial infarction

By Harald Sanne, Dag Elmfeldt and Lars Wilhelmsen

There is so far no proof of any preventive effect of physical exercise on coronary heart disease, neither primary nor secondary. Some authors claim a benefical effect (4, 5) but there are no controlled studies of a randomized, respresentative series.

However, there are many observations which have brought attention to this possibility. In the early fifties Morris observed the difference in incidence of coronary heart disease in sedentary and physically active workers (9). Since then many population studies have confirmed this fact (for ref. see 13). Eckstein has shown experimental evidence of physical training as a way of increasing the collateral dimensions in obstructed coronary vessels in dogs (2). Physical training will give a reduction of triglycerides and possibly also of blood cholesterol (1, 6, 7, 8, 14).

All these observations have raised expectations and induced some feasibility studies (4, 5, 8, 10). Remington and co-workers have estimated the proportions of a series necessary to prove any preventive effect (11). They conclude the need of large groups of subjects, the number being dependent on several factors such as death rates, size of preventive effect, adherence to the programs, etc.

This is a preliminary report of a secondary preventive study with physical training. Till now, the time of follow up is short, on a average 1.9 years. Mortality and reinfarction rate in this series is reported. The study has a broader aspect examining the training effect on angina pectoris, physical working capacity, the patients spontaneous physical activity, metabolism and other variables.

Patient series and methods

The patients come from the city of Göteborg with 450 000 inhabitants. The series consists of all patients born in 1913 and later who suffered an acute myocardial infarction (MI) during 1968, 1969 and 1970 and were discharged from hospital alive.

In Göteborg there is one main hospital for the acute care of patients. An Ischaemic Heart Disease Register is working in the city. Some cases of MI will however, not be discovered. Some patients may be treated at

Table 1. *Effect of physical training.*

Myocardial infarction patients, born 1913 and later, living in Göteborg, who became ill during the years 1968–1970.

Total number		316	
Randomized to	Training 156		Control 160
Surviving 3 months	151		153
Started training	111		0
Mean follow up time (yrs.)	1.85		1.85
Mortality before 30.6.71:			
Total	18		26
Due to CHD	15		25
Mortality 26 weeks after MI and later:			
Total	8	$p<0.05$	19
Due to CHD	6	$p<0.025$	18

home and not discovered but according to a study in 1968 there are practically no diagnosed MIs taken care of at home. If a patient from Göteborg suffer a MI outside the city he will usually be sent to the Sahlgren's Hospital and registered. Thus, we consider this series of MI patients representative.

After discharge from hospital all patients are treated and followed up at a special post-MI clinic. This organization makes it possible to give a uniform treatment and perform a standardized follow up program (3).

Three months after the MI all patients are called to a special examination including serum lipids, a heart *X*-ray and an ergometer test. The latter is performed on a bicycle and repeated after some days in order to find out the patients highest physical capacity and limiting factors to this performance.

When registered during the hospital stay the patients are randomized with the aid of a random number table into one training group and one control group. The patients are considered to belong to these original groups during the whole follow up period. Thus, the training group is defined by the randomization and not by attendance or trainability. On the other hand, some patients in the control group will definitely take part in various physical training programs but will still be considered as controls.

After the MI all patients are given general recommendations about gradually increased physical strain during the convalescense period and they are requested to take walks. There is nowadays rather much attention paid to physical activity in the population, and we find that about 10 % of the control patients have an own training bicycle for use indoors.

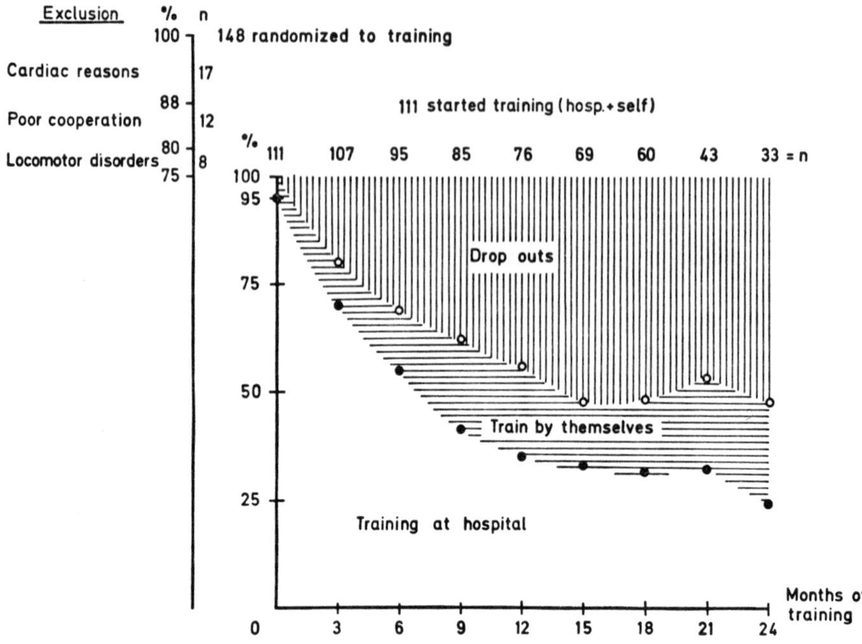

Fig. 1. Primary exclusion and secondary drop out rate of 148 patients randomized to training.

The training program consists of three sessions, of 30 minutes each, every week (13). The exercises are mainly dynamic, involving large muscle groups in order to load the heart and central circulation. The intensity is regulated by a physiotherapist with the use of the heart rate (12). On an average the highest heart rate measured during training has been about 10 beats lower than the highest tolerated heart rate during the ergometer test.

The training team has not been involved in the ordinary medical treatment of the patients.

Results

The number of patients with MI who fit the definition born in 1913 and later, living in Göteborg, and falling ill during the years 1968 through 1970, was 316. The training group consisted of 156 cases and the control group of 160. In these two groups, 151 and 153 cases, respectively, survived the first three months (Table 1). One hundred and fourtyeight patients in the training group were tested on bicycle ergometer and evaluated before training (Fig. 1). Thirtyseven patients or 25 per cent were excluded

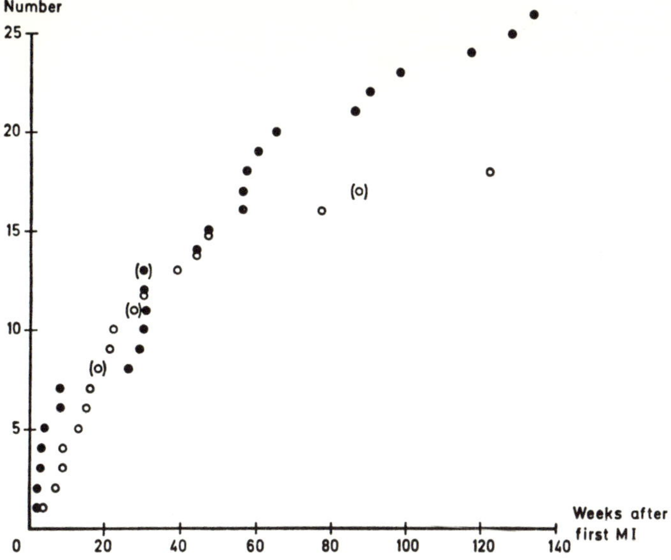

Fig. 2. Accumulated number of deaths in the original groups randomized to training and to control. Brackets denote deaths due to other reasons than coronary heart disease.

—the largest group because of cardiac reasons, 12 per cent. One hundred and eleven patients started training.

There was a high rate of drop-out. After two years, only 25 per cent of those who started were still training at the hospital. Further 25 per cent were training independently but still under direction. They had got the opportunity to use an ergometer bicycle at home or at their place of work. They used an individually prescribed program and their physical working capacity was regularly checked.

Figure 2 shows the accumulated deaths, from coronary disease as well as from other disease in the two groups until June 1971.

The death rate was equal in the two groups during the first year. Then there was a difference. Statistical analysis of the total deaths in the two groups during the follow-up period gave no difference. The number of deaths were 18 and 26 respectively (Table 1). However, as training was not offered until about 15 weeks after the MI any effect could hardly be expected before this time. There was no statistical difference between the groups in number of deaths 15 weeks after the MI and later. However, we consider that the training has to go on for some time before any effect can be expected. Therefore, the death rate was calculated from 6 months (26 weeks) after the MI to the end of the follow-up period. During this period there were 8 deaths in the training group and 19 in the control

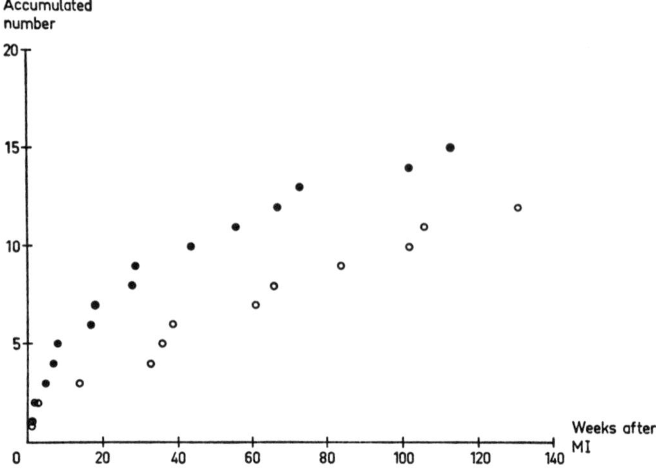

Fig. 3. Accumulated number of reinfarctions in the original groups randomized to training and to control.

group. The difference is significant at the 5 per cent level according to chi-squared test.

Figure 3 shows the accumulated number of reinfarctions during the follow-up period. There was no statistical difference between the two groups. Only one reinfarction was recorded in each patient and no reinfarction in patients who died.

Comments

This preliminary report has shown that relative intense physical training can be carried out in a non-selected series of MI patients. In this age group, however, 25 per cent could not start training, the main reason being cardiac contraindications. Although the patients are enthusiastic at the beginning, the rate of drop out is high especially during the initial stage. When the patients are back to work they have practical difficulties in continuing the training at the hospital dependent on long travelling, lack of time, inconvenient time for training although they have been offered training sessions early in the mornings and after work.

Patients with low working tolerance and no effect of the training had higher drop out rate. Many other motivational factors seem to interfere with the patients cooperation. Some do not like to visit a hospital, others think the training reminds them of the MI and increase their feeling ill. The adherence is of course dependent on geographical and local circumstances.

The results indicate that this type of training is not dangerous to the patients. There has, however, been one accident with ventricular fibrillation during a training session. The patient was resuscitated and is still alive and working full time. Apart from this occasion the reinfarctions and deaths have not occurred in relation to training or exercise testing.

The results til now suggest a secondary preventive effect of this therapy. The project will proceed, keeping the two groups separated. Symptoms and signs, physical working capacity, and ECG-signs during exercise, blood lipids, blood coagulation and fibrinolysis, and some other variables are continously followed in the two groups.

References

1. Dalderup, L. M., De Voogd, N., Meyknecht, E. A. M. & Den Hartog, C.: The effects of increasing the daily physical activity on the serum cholesterol levels. *Nutr. Dieta 9:* 112, 1967.
2. Eckstein, R. W.: Effect of exercise and coronary artery narrowing on coronary collateral circulation. *Circ. Res. 5:* 230, 1957.
3. Elmfeldt, D. & Wilhelmsen, L.: A study of representative postmyocardial infarction patients aged 25–55. Se pp. 129, this volume.
4. Gottheiner, V.: Long-range strenous sports training for cardiac reconditioning an rehabilitation. *Amer. J. Cardiol. 22:* 426, 1968.
5. Hellerstein, H. K.: The effects of physical activity. Patients and normal coronary prone subjects. *Minn. Med. 52:* 1335, 1969.
5. Holloszy, J. O., Skinner, J. S., Toro, G. & Cureton, T. K.: Effects of a six months program of endurance exercise on the serum lipids of middle-aged men. *Amer. J. Cardiol. 14:* 753, 1964.
7. Kilbom, Å., Hartley, L. H., Saltin, B., Bjure, J., Grimby, G. & Åstrand, I.: Physical training in sedentary middle aged and older men. I. Medical evaluation. *Scand. J. Clin. Lab. Invest. 24:* 315, 1969.
8. Mann, G. V., Garrett, H. L., Fahri, A., Murray, H., Billings, F. T. Shute. F. & Schwarten, S. E.: Exercise to prevent coronary heart disease. *Amer. J. Med. 46*: 12, 1969.
9. Morris, J., Heady, J., Raffle, P., Roberts, C. & Parks, J.: Coronary heart disease and physical activity of work. *Lancet ii:* 1053, 1111, 1953.
10. Pyörälä, K., Käräva, R., Punsar, S., Oja, P., Teräslinna, P., Partanen, T., Jääskeläinen, M., Pekkarinen, M.-L. & Koskela, A.: A controlled study of the effects of 18 months' physical training in sedentary middle-aged men with high indexes of risk relative to coronary heart disease. In *Coronary heart disease and physical fitness*. Munksgaard, Copenhagen, 1971.
11. Remington, R. & Schork, M. A.: Determination of number of subjects needed for experimental epidemiologic studies of the effect of increased physical activity on incidence of coronary heart–disease–preliminary considerations. *Physical activity and the heart*. Thomas, Springfield, Ill., 1967.

12. Rydin, C. E. & Sanne, H.: On the possibility to direct a safe physical training program for coronary diseased patients. *Scand. J. Rehab. Med.*, 1971.
13. Sanne, H. M. & Wilhelmsen, L.: Physical activity as prevention and therapy in coronary heart disease. *Scand J. Rehab. Med. 3:* 47, 1971.
14. Siegel, W., Blomqvist, G. & Mitchell, J. H.: Effects of a quantitated physical training program on middle-aged sedentary men. *Circulation 41:* 19, 1970.

This investigation was supported by a grant from Förenade Liv, Stockholm.

Evaluation of a myocardial infarction out-patient clinic — A Secondary Preventive Trial

By J. Anders Vedin and Claes E. Wilhelmsson

In Gothenburg since 1968, patients with myocardial infarction below 57 years of age have been taken care of in a special out-patient clinic for post-hospital care and follow-up (1). Since January 1st, 1970, patients with myocardial infarction, between 57 and 67 years of age, have been included in another out-patient clinic. This programme is designed to study two major problems:

a) The effects of a post-hospital MI clinic
b) The effects of chornic beta-receptor inhibition after myocardial infarction.

The patients are identified by the WHO registry in Gothenburg and patients with myocardial infarction according to the WHO criteria are accepted for study (2).

In order to establish the possibble effects of an out-patient clinic all male patients, born on dates ending with 3, 6 and 9, are allocated to the control group. This group is managed entirely outside the present project and the patients are not seen by the project personnel.

The patients follow the routine follow-up schedule outlined in Figure 1.

Throughout the study efforts are made to control interobserver variation. Standardized procedures are used together with data records using previously validated questionnaires on chest pain, angina pectoris, breathlessness, cardiac decompensation etc. Unambiguous criteria are used for treatment of symptoms, signs, risk factors and complications. In the study, efforts are made to provide maximal interaction between nurse and patient. The patients are instructed to consult the study personnel whenever needed. They are first seen at the clinic within one week after discharge from hospital. The first visit is devoted to the introduction of the patient to the clinic and to the completion of medical history and a physical examination.

In Figure 1 at the visits marked with an asterisk, the patients are seen by one of the two physicians of the project. At the remaining visits the patients are interviewed by a specially trained nurse also measuring blood pressure and taking blood samples.

11 – 729766 *Tibblin m. fl.*

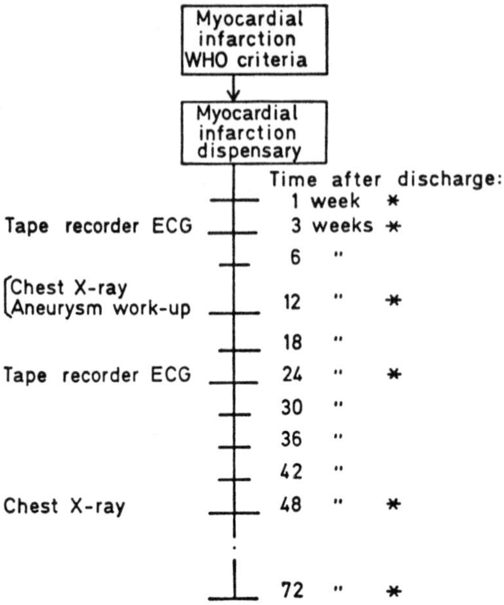

Fig. 1. Routine follow-up schedule for patients with myocardial infarction, 57–67 years of age. Examination by physician.

The results of the clinic evaluation and the beta-receptor inhibitor trial are evaluated in homogenous subgroups. The criteria for the allocation of patients to the subgroups were obtained from the study of younger myocardial infarction patients below correlated to death or reinfarction during the first year of follow-up (1969) (3). For convenience, the criteria were grouped as follows: I. lack of extensive cardiac damage, II. mechanical cardiac damage, III. electrical damage and IV. combined electro-mechanical damage to the heart. This is illustrated in Figure 2. The presence of one single factor was sufficient for allocation to a specific subgroup. The following end-points were used: a) death from any cause, 2) coronary death, 3) non-fatal reinfarction.

Reinfarctions and deaths in the clinic control groups are monitored by the WHO registry. Routine hospital records of this group are checked annually. In the experimental group changing frequencies of angina pectoris and dyspnoea are studied together with time fluctuations of the coronary risk factors. Special attention is paid to arrhythmias studied at intervals throughout the post-hospital period. Tape recorders and a system of computer analysis are used permitting the evaluation of long term recordings. In a particular study efforts are made to correlate clinical data and results from physical and plain *X*-ray examination with data from catheterization and angiographic examinations on patients with left ventricular aneurysms (Figur 1).

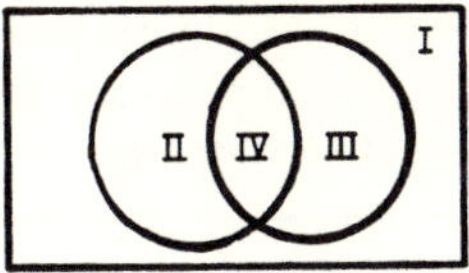

Sub-group I: No extensive cardiac damage

Sub-group II: Mechanical damage to myocardium

1) Rel. heart volume ♂ >450 ml/m² BSA; ♀ >400 ml/m² BSA

2) GPT >40 U during first 3 days

3) BT >38 °C " " " "

4) Transient atrial flutter and fibrillation

Sub-group III: Electrical cardiac damage

1) VPB frequency >5/min

2) Ventricular tachycardia or ventricular fibrillation

3) AV-blocks: a. PQ > 0.24 s; b. Type II; c. Type III

Sub-group IV: Combined electro-mechanical damage (Sub-groups II o. III)

Fig. 2. Criteria for homogenous sub-group allocation of patients with myocardial infarction, 57–67 years of age.

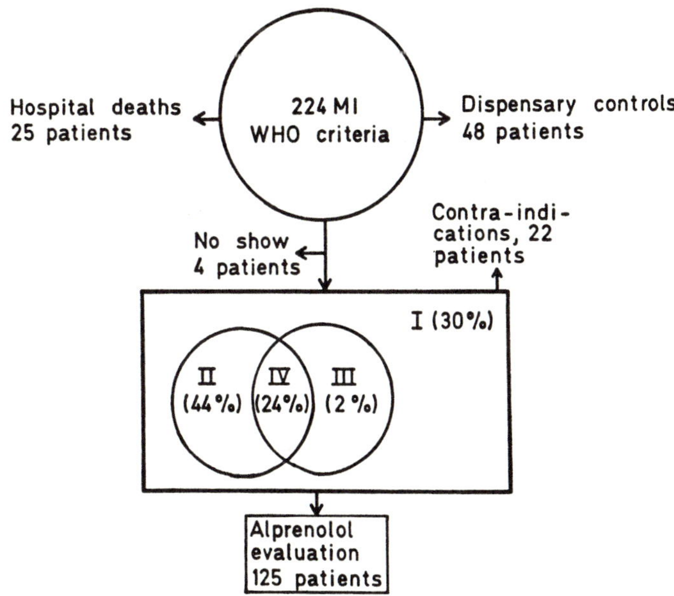

Fig. 3. Patients with myocardial infarction, 57–67 years of age, 1970 cohort.

Table 1. Out-patient clinic evaluation, 1970 cohort. Mortality and reinfarction among male patients with myocardial infarction, 57–67 years of age in experimental and control groups. Average follow-up period: 7.5 months.

	Clinic patients	Controls
Deaths	9	8
%	9	16
Reinfarction	7	9
%	7	18
Total number of patients	103	48

After exclusion of patients with contra-indications to beta-receptor antagonists the patients of each subgroup are randomly allocated to placebo or active treatment with alprenolol 400 mg daily. The end points and variables of this part of the study are identical to those mentioned above.

Patients will continuously be admitted to the programmes for two years (1970–1971) and the follow-up time will be 18 months.

During the first year, 1970, 224 patients between 57 and 67 years of age fulfilling the criteria of myocardial infarction, were accepted for the study (Figure 3). During the first year 48 patients were allocated to the control group.

The present presentation is confined to some results based on the patients collected during 1970 and followed for an average period of 7.5 months.

Twenty-two patients presenting contra-indications to beta-blocking agents, were excluded from this part of the study but were maintained in the out-patient clinic evaluation. Ten of these patients needed continuous medication for chronic obstructive pulmonary disease, five were suffering from severe hypotension and seven could not participate for phycho-social reasons. Five of these were chronic alcoholics. Only four patients entirely refused to co-operate during the first year. Thus 125 patients remained to enter the drug trial. The proportions of patients in the four subgroups are shown in Figure 3. Patients with ventricular arrhythmias without extensive mechanical damage were rare in this post-hospital population. The major part of patients having had arrhythmias also had signs of extensive cardiac damage and were referred to group IV.

During the follow-up period 16 non-fatal myocardial infarctions and 17 coronary deaths were recorded. Out of nine deaths in the experimental group six occurred in subgroup IV, one in subgroup III and two in sub-group II. The distribution of these events in the experimental and the control group is shown in Table 1. Thus, these subgroups provide a means of isolating high and low risk patients with regard to mortality. It should be noted that the mortality of the contra-indications group is high with 7 deaths (men and women) out of 22 subjects or around 30 per cent.

The demonstrated difference in rates of death and reinfarction between the patients treated at the clinic and the controls do not permit far reaching conclusions due to insufficient size of the groups. It is not explained by alprenolol effects (4). However, the trend justifies continued studies into secondary prevention by means of a specialized out-patient clinic.

References

1. Elmfelt, D. & Wilhelmsen, L.: Hjärtinfarkt – morbiditet, mortalitet och invaliditet. *Läkartidningen 68:* 3705–3710, 1971.
2. Fodor, J. & Tibblin, G.: One year's experience of the work of the Ischemic Heart Disease Registry in Gothenburg in Ischemic Heart Disease Registers. Report of the Fourth Working Group, Copenhagen, WHO Regional Office for Europe, 1970.
3. Wilhelmsen, L.: Personal communication, 1969.
4. Wilhelmsson, C. & Vedin, A.: A preventive trial with alprenolol after myocardial infarction. Preliminary results from the first 18 months. The III Scandinavian Congress of Cardiology, Helsinki, Finland, 1971.

Lipoprotein pattern in IHD

By Gösta Dahlén, Curt Ericson,
Curt Furberg, Lennart Lundkvist
and Kurt Svärdsudd

Ten months ago a screening population study among 40–60 years old men was started in the Boden area in northern Sweden. The Gothenburg design was used in this multifactor preventive trial that had in view to identify subjects with high IHD risk and to modify the risk factors. It was found to interest to include electrophoresis of lipoproteins in the serum lipid analyzes to get an idea about its value in this type of population study.

The material in this presentation includes 311 men between the ages of 56 to 60 years with completed lipid analyzes.

A postal questionary dealing with different habits and cardiovascular disease was sent to the subjects. An abbreviated version of the London School of Hygiene Cardiovascular questionnaire was used to detect subjects with symptoms of angina of effort.

Among those who answered the questionary every second man was invited to a medical examination which included blood sampling for chemical analyzes. These examinations were usually carried out in the afternoon for practical reasons. The subjects were asked not to eat within 4 to 6 hours before the examination. Electrophoresis of lipoproteins was performed with cellogel Sepraphore III as supporting medium. All subjects who answered that they got precordial pain of discomfort when they walked uphill or hurried were interviewed for clinical judgement of the symptoms.

During preliminary work with the results it was soon noted that patients with symptoms of angina of effort often had an extra electrophoretic fraction between the beta and pre-beta bands. We have named this fraction the pre-beta-1 fraction. Sixty-four subjects in all or about 20 % of the material had a detectable pre-beta-1 in the electrophoresis (Figs. 1 and 2).

Seventy-one men out of 311 answered in the questionary that they got precordial pain or discomfort in the chest when they walked uphill or hurried. Twenty-four men in this group had a pre-beta-1 fraction. There was a highly statistical correlation between a positive answer to this question and the occurrence of a pre-beta-1 fraction (Fig. 3). Fifty-two men out of these 71 were judged as cases with typical or suspect angina of effort and 20 out of them had this extra lipoprotein fraction. The correlation

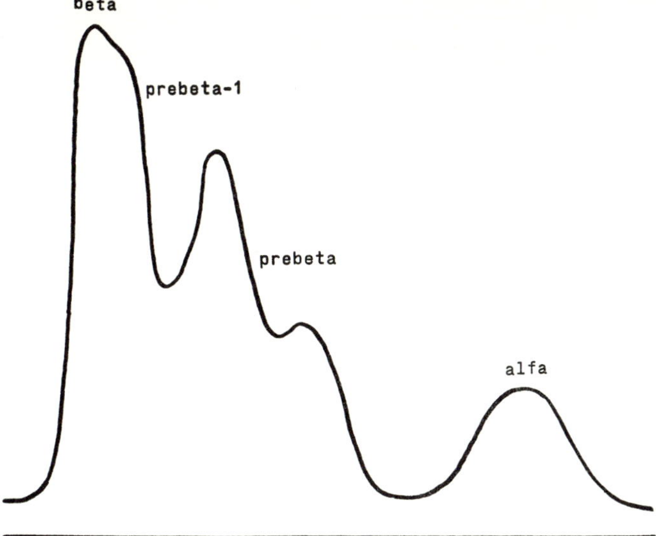

Fig. 1. A prominent pre-beta-1 fraction.

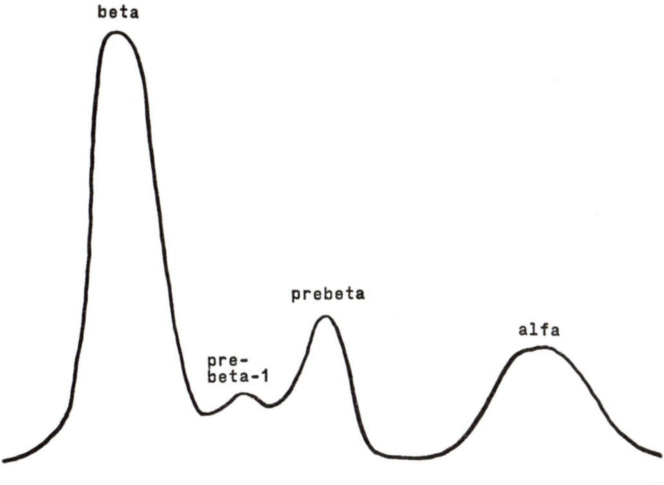

Fig. 2. A small pre-beta-1 fraction.

		Pre-beta-1 +	Pre-beta-1 −	
Do you get any pain or discomfort in your chest when you walk uphill or hurry?	+	24	47	71
	−	40	200	240
		64	247	311

$p < 0.01$

Fig. 3. The correlation between chest pain according to the questionary and the occurrence of a pre-beta-1 fraction.

		Pre-beta-1 +	Pre-beta-1 −	
Typical or suspected AP among those who answered that they got pain when walking uphill or hurrying.	+	20	32	52
	−	44	215	259
		64	247	311

$p < 0.001$

Fig. 4. The correlation between clinical diagnosis of angina of effort and the occurrence of a pre-beta-1 fraction.

between the clinical diagnosis of angina of effort and the occurrence of a pre-beta-1 fraction was also statistically highly significant (Fig. 4).

This piling up of subjects with symptoms of angina of effort among those with pre-beta-1 gave rise to a reexamination of all subjects with this fraction and no precordial pain when walking uphill according to the questionary. The diagnoses of the 64 men with pre-beta-1 after this re-examination are shown in Fig. 5. About two thirds of these men had symptoms or signs of heart disease.

The pre-beta-1 fraction was detectable about twice as often in men with high cholesterol and/or triglycerides compared to those with normal serum lipids. This number is somewhat uncertain as the pre-beta-1 sometimes is difficult to detect in combination with a broad pre-beta band. Fig. 6 shows the electrophoretic pattern in a man before and after diet therapy.

Diagnosis	
Typical angina of effort	15
Suspect angina of effort	13
Cardiac decompensation	1
Atypical chest symptoms	7
Arrhythmia cordis	3
Untreated art. hypertension	3
No symptoms and signs of heart disease	22
	$n = 64$

Fig. 5. The diagnoses of 64 men between the ages of 56 to 60 years with a pre-beta-1 fraction.

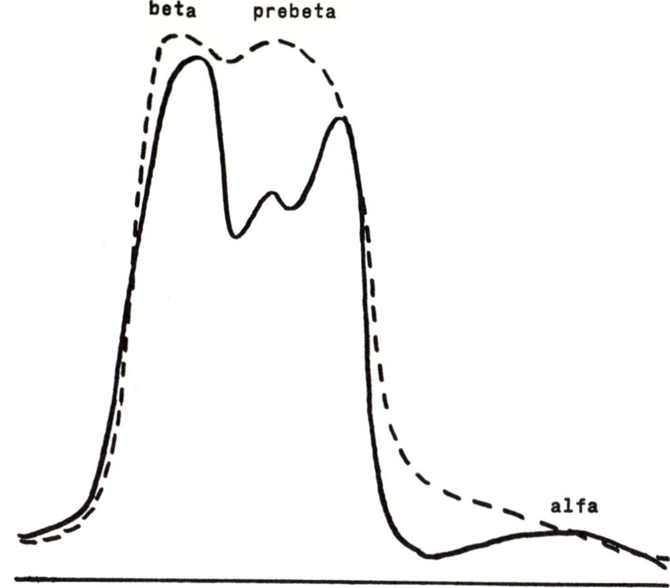

Fig. 6. The electrophoretic pattern in a man before (short dashes) and after diet therapy.

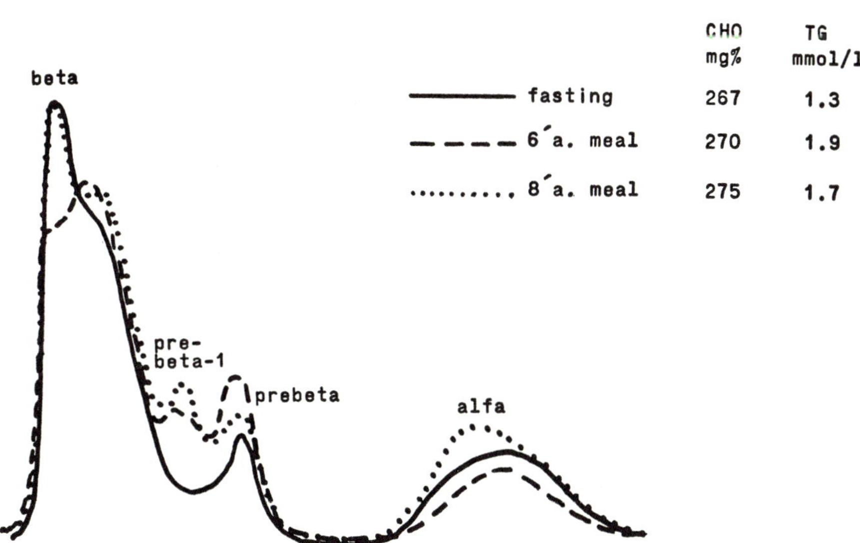

Fig. 7. The electrophoretic patterns before, 6 and 8 hours after a test meal in a patient with angina of effort.

	n	age	+	suspect	–
MI	20*	47–65	9	2	7
AP	6	56–60	5	1	0
Controls	10	56–60	2	1	7
Controls	13	21–46	3	0	10

* see text

Fig. 8. Detectable, suspect and not detectable pre-beta-1 fraction respectively 8 hours after a test meal in patients with myocardial infarction (MI) and angina of effort (AP) and in healthy control subjects.

During tests to reproduce the pre-beta-1 fraction it sometimes occurred that this fraction was not detectable in samples taken overnight fasting especially in those with low triglycerides. Serial analyzes have shown that the pre-beta-1 fraction is often best seen in the afternoon 6 to 8 hours after a given test meal (Fig. 7).

We have studied the effect of a test meal on the electrophoretic pattern in different groups of patients and in healthy control subjects (Fig. 8). Ten out of the 20 patients with a history of myocardial infarction had elevated serum lipids. Two out of these cases had a broad pre-beta band that made the interpretation of the electrophoresis concerning pre-beta-1 impossible. Nine of the remaining 18 patients had a detectable pre-beta-1 fraction 8 hours after a test meal and two cases had a suspect extra fraction. Another 7 had no detectable extra fraction after the test meal. A pre-beta-1 fraction was found in five out of 23 healthy subjects in different age groups 8 hours after a test meal.

Besides a genetic factor seems to influence the appearance of the pre-beta-1 fraction (Fig. 9).

Our electrophoretic studies have given interesting results. It is too early to comment on the correlation between the pre-beta-1 fraction and heart disease. It seems as if electrophoresis of lipoproteins is of value in screening population studies among middle-aged or older men to identify subjects with symptoms and signs of heart disease.

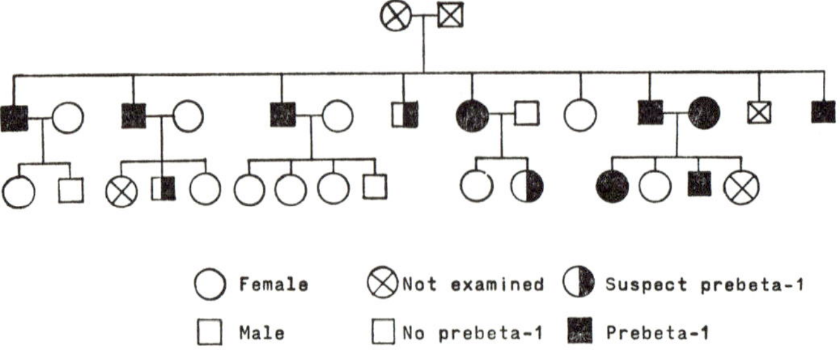

Fig. 9. The pedigree of a family with a high number of subjects with a pre-beta-1 fraction.

Calf blood flow and smoking

By Sven-Olof Isacsson

Jean Nicot, French ambassador to Lisbon, after whom nicotine was named, recommended the use of tobacco in the belief that it was salutary. Today, however, we know that the habit of smoking is not conductive to health, but harmful. Relatively recent investigations have produced strong evidence of a connection between smoking, morbidity and mortality in several diseases, including ischemic heart disease. Furthermore, observations on record suggest that smoking favours not only ischemic heart disease, but also the development of generalized atherosclerosis (1, 2). Investigations of the connection between smoking and arteriosclerotic diseases should therefore not be confined to ischemic heart disease. In the enormous epidemiologic research in cardiovascular diseases during the last two decades very little attention has been given to diseases of the peripheral arteries. It might therefore not be out of place to quote G. Schettler's introductory lecture at the Second International Symposium on Atherosclerosis: »What are the problems we should deal with in the future? As a clinician I would like to mention a few points. Epidemiology should focus not only on coronary heart disease but also on other vascular areas and should use all the available diagnostic tools. The risk factors in atherogenesis will have different weights in different vascular areas.» (3).

Smoking is considered one of the most potent risk-factors for ischemic heart disease, independent of all other risk factors (4, 5).

In this population study the calf blood flow in both legs was determined routinely with venous occlusion plethysmography. The results thus obtained were related to smoking and other data collected in connection with the population study.

Material and methods

In 1969 an epidemiologic cross-sectional study was carried out in Malmö (260 000 inhabitants), Sweden, regarding the prevalence of cardiovascular and lung diseases. Full participation was obtained from 703 (87 %) of 809 randomly selected men born in 1914 and residing in Malmö at the time of the study. Out of these 703 men, 684 were examined with venous occlusion plethysmography. Seventeen refused to undergo this examination. These persons did not differ in any other respect from the rest of the material.

Table 1. Procedure of examination. Men born in 1914. N = 703.

1. Questionnaire, regarding angina pectoris, intermittent claudication (12), smoking habits etc.
2. Blood pressure
3. Physical examination
4. Weight and height
5. Cholesterol, triglycerides, haematocrit
6. Spirometry
7. Electrocardiogram
8. Chest *X*-ray (determination of heart volume)
9. Calf blood flow (venous occlusion plethysmography)

The examination procedures is presented in Table 1.

The examinations were performed between 7 a.m. and 11 a.m. The subjects were instructed not to eat or smoke after midnight previous to the examination. They were divided into three groups according to their smoking habits:

1. "Never-smoked"; (less than 1 cigarette a day for less than a year).
2. Ex-smokers, consisting of those who had stopped smoking at least one month before the examination.
3. Smokers, consisting of inhalers as well as non-inhalers.

The number of cigarettes smoked per day was expressed as grams of tobacco, one cigarette being taken as 1 gram of tobacco, one cheroot as two grams and one cigar as five grams. The consumption of pipe tobacco was given in grams per day (24 hours) as was the total consumption of tobacco. The smokers were then divided into three groups, corresponding to daily consumption of 1–14, 15–24 and 25 grams or more.

The calf blood flow was measured with venous occlusion plethysmography with a water-filled system. The apparatus and technique were essentially the same as those described by Dahn (11). By occluding the arterial inflow to the limbs for 3 minutes by cuffs wrapped around the thighs, reactive hyperaemia was produced on release of the occlusion (8, 9). During the reactive hyperemia the vascular bed distal to the cuff is considered to be almost maximally dilated. Reduced flow during reactive hyperaemia occurs mainly in presence of conditions restricting the lumen of the arterial tree (8). It has been shown that the first flow measured during reactive hyperaemia is the parameter that best discriminates between individuals with and without arterial disease (13). The classification of the population in this study was therefore based on the first flow during reactive hyperaemia. This flow was, however, observed to be significantly correlated to the systolic and diastolic arm blood pressure measured during the plethysmographic recording, and even with the pulse rate. Furthermore, a negative correlation was found between first flow and standing

Table 2. *Smoking habits in the population. N=703.*

	Never smoked	Ex-smokers	Smokers inhalers	Smokers non-inhalers	All smokers	Total consumption of tobacco g/day 1–14	15–24	≥25
Number	108	159	77	359	436	258	141	37
Per cent of the population	15	23	11	51	63	37	20	5

height. In order to make the subjects comparable, the influence of these factors on the first flow was mathematically accounted for. A new variable was calculated for each subject and referred to as *flow capacity*.

Flow capacity was calculated in the following way:

$$\left(\frac{\textit{observed first flow}}{\textit{predicted first flow}} \times 100\right).$$

In this way a percental value was obtained. The predicted first flow was calculated with the aid of multiple regression analysis as follows:

Predicted first flow=(pulse rate×0.05)+(mean blood pressure×0.10)−(height×0.18)+38.33.

The mean blood pressure was calculated from the diastolic arm blood pressure plus one third of the pulse pressure. It was thus possible to compare the observed first flow in each subject with his predicted first flow. A flow capacity of 100 % thus corresponds to the mean value for the entire population. The lower the flow capacity, the stronger the reason to suspect arteriosclerotic disease.

Results

The smoking habits of the population are outlined in Table 2. 62.3 % of the selected men were smokers. Analysis of the previous smoking habits of the ex-smokers showed that the ex-smokers had started smoking at the same age as those who were still smoking, i.e. approximately at the age of 19, and that they had smoked until an average age of 43. Consequently, the ex-smokers had not smoked for, on the average, 12 years prior to the examination. The ex-smokers had previously consumed as much tobacco as those who were still smoking at the time of study.

Relation between smoking habits and flow capacity

In Figure 1 the material is divided into deciles of the flow capacity and the prevalence of different smoking habits is given for each decile. Each

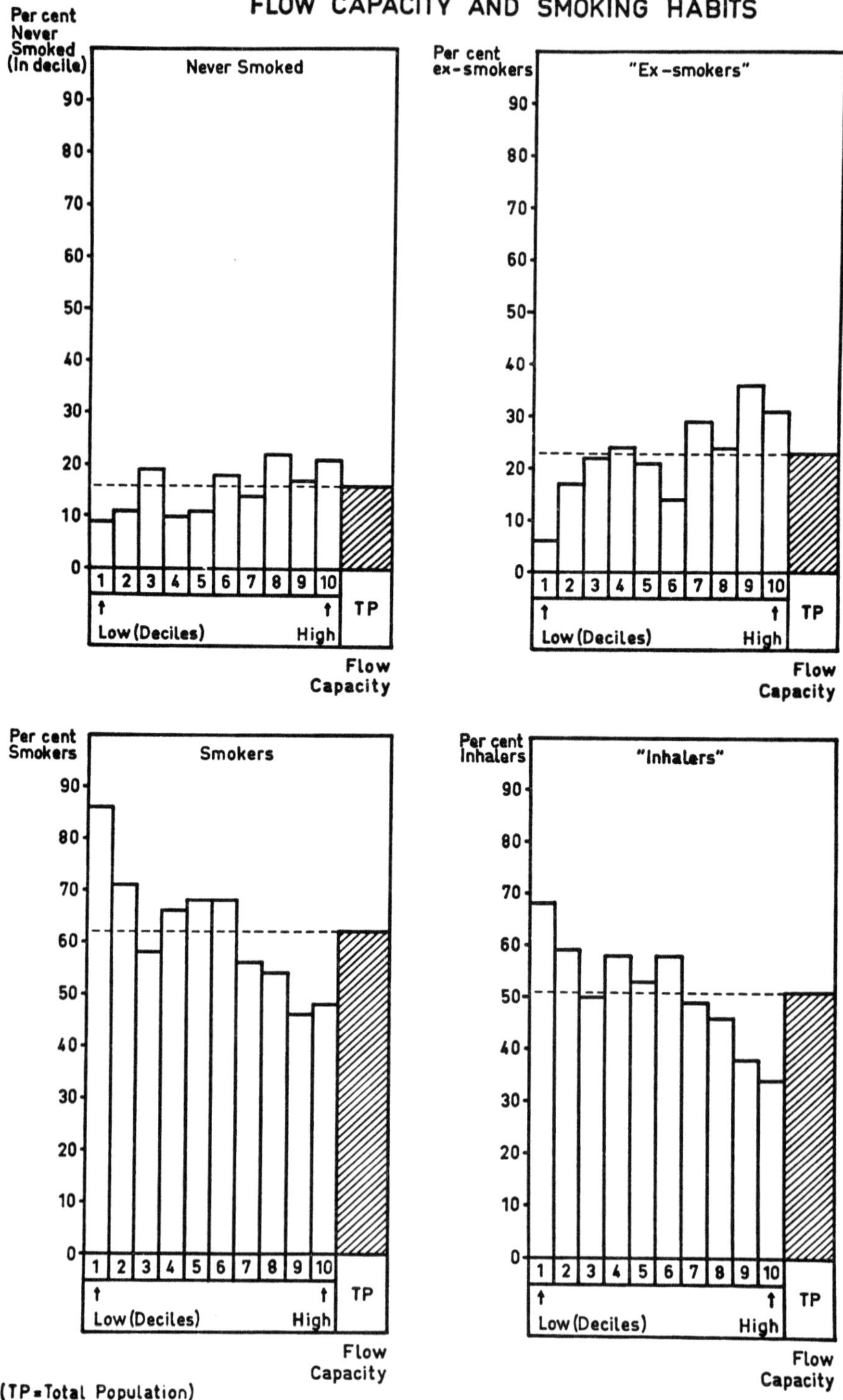

Fig. 1. Smoking habits in different deciles of the flow capacity.

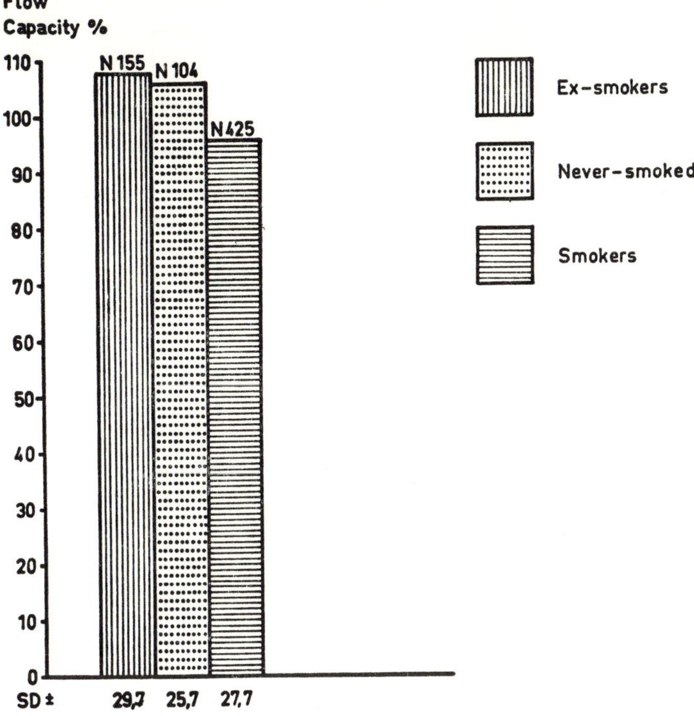

Fig. 2. Smoking habits and flow capacity.

decile has been compared with the entire material. For those who had never smoked, no significant difference was found between the different deciles and the material as a whole. The ex-smokers were significantly fewer ($p < 0.01$) in the first decile. Furthermore, the total number of smokers was significantly larger ($p < 0.001$) in decile 1, and smaller ($p < 0.05$) in the two highest deciles. There were more subjects who inhaled the smoke in the first decile ($p < 0.05$) and fewer in the two highest deciles (decile 9 $p < 0.05$, decile 10 $p < 0.01$).

The relation between flow capacity and the smoking habits, is given in Figures 2, 3 and 4. Figure 2 shows that the ex-smokers had a higher flow capacity than those who had never smoked, but the difference was not statistically significant. The flow capacity among the smokers, regardless of their daily consumption of tobacco, was significantly lower than

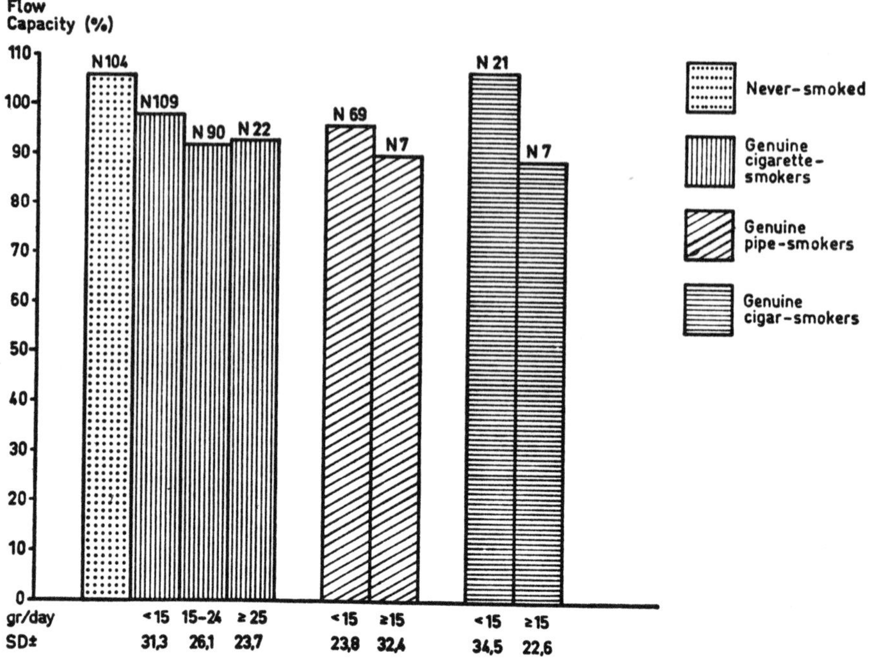

Fig. 3. Smoking habits and flow capacity.

among those who had never smoked ($p < 0.01$). Many smokers were cigarette-, pipe- and cigarsmokers. These subjects are not included in Figure 3, which embraces only genuine cigarette smokers, pipe smokers or cigar smokers. In smokers with a cigarette consumption of 15 gram or more per day the flow capacity was significantly lower ($p < 0.001$) than among those who had never smoked. The flow capacity among pipe smokers consuming 1–14 grams per day, was significantly lower than among those who had never smoked ($p < 0.01$). In the few pipe smokers (7), who consumed 15 grams or more a day the flow capacity was as low as that of heavy cigarette smokers. Finally, Figure 4 gives the size of the flow capacity in relation to the total daily consumption. At a consumption of 1–14 grams per day, the flow capacity was slightly lower than that in those who had never smoked ($p < 0.05$). In those smoking 15 grams or more a day, the flow capacity was significantly reduced ($p < 0.001$). There was no further reduction in those smoking more than 25 grams a day.

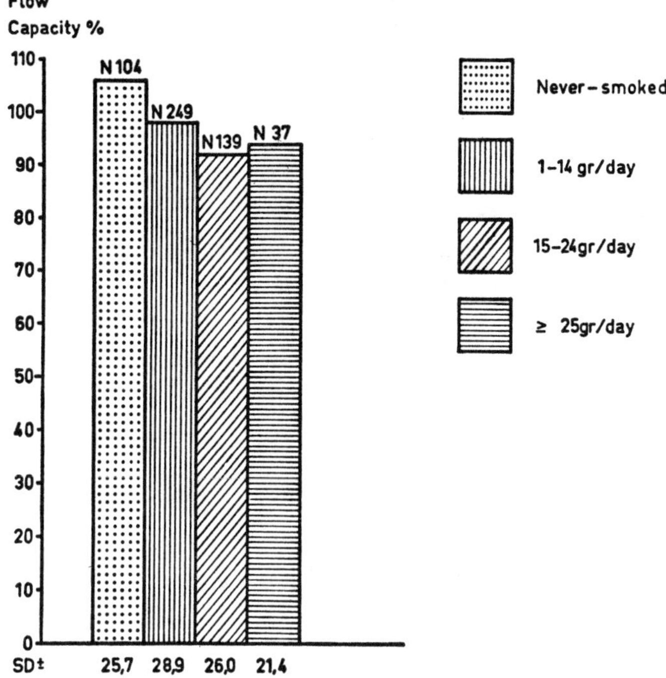

Fig. 4. Smoking habits and flow capacity.

Discussion

Autopsy studies have shown that smoking promotes the development of atherosclerosis in the entire arterial system (1, 2). This might reflect an atherogenic effect of carbon monoxide (6, 7). The flow capacity was calculated from the first flow during reactive hyperaemia, and investigations carried out by other authors have clearly shown that the release of 3 minutes' occlusion of the arterial inflow to the extremities is followed by an almost maximal dilatation of the arterial bed (8, 9). The reductions of flow capacity observed in this study may therefore be taken as evidence of a process reducing the arterial lumen, and at the age of this population, organic changes in the arteries consist mainly of atherosclerosis (14).

This study did not reveal any other factor capable of explaining the relatively low flow capacity in the smokers. It is true that the first flow during reactive hyperaemia, *i.e.* the variable on which the calculation of flow capacity was based, was significantly correlated with arm blood pressure, pulse rate and height. But the calculation of flow capacity implied that the influence of these factors on the first flow was eliminated. Furthermore, it should be stressed that the smokers, probably, with a few exceptions, had not smoked for 6–7 hours before the examination. This study suggests that the reduction in flow capacity varies with the consumption of tobacco per day, independently of the fact whether the tobacco is consumed in the form of cigarettes, pipe-tobacco or cigars. It is, however, apparent that real pipe smokers or cigar smokers are rarely heavy smokers, if consumption of 15 grams tobacco or more per day can be regarded as sufficient to classify a person as a heavy smoker. On the whole, it seems to be of no importance what one smokes, but how much one smokes. This agrees well with the findings in recent investigations that the cigar and pipe smokers smoking large amounts of tobacco per day and inhaling the smoke, run essentially the same risk of getting coronary heart disease as the heavy smokers of cigarettes (10).

Conclusions

The results of this study show that the arterial flow capacity in the calf calculated from the first flow during reactive hyperaemia, was reduced in the smokers and that this reduction was greatest in the inhalers and in the heavy smokers, *i.e.* those smoking 15 grams a day or more. The reduced flow capacity of the smokers is considered a probable cause of structural arterial changes, probably arteriosclerosis.

References

1. Sackett, D. L., Gibson, R. W., Bross, I. D. J. & Pickren, J. W.: Relation between aortic atherosclerosis and the use of cigarettes and alcohol. An autopsy study. *New Engl. J. Med. 279*: 1413, 1968.
2. Auerbach, O., Hammond, C. & Garfinkel, L.: Thickening of walls of arterioles and small arteries in relation to age and smoking habits. *New Engl. J. Med. 278:* 980, 1968.
3. Schettler, G.: In Atherosclerosis: *Proceedings of the Second International Symposium.* Springer-Verlag, Berlin. New York, 1970.
4. Morris, J. N., Kagan, A., Pattison, D. C., Gardner, M. J. & Raffle, P. A. B.: Incidence and prediction of ischaemic heart disease in London busmen. *Lancet 2*: 553, 1966.
5. Truett, J., Cornfield, J. & Kannel, W.: A multivariate analysis of the risk of coronary heart disease in Framingham, *J. Chron. Dis. 20*: 511, 1967.
6. Astrup, P., Kjeldsen, K. & Wanstrup, J.: Enhancing influence of carbon monoxide on the development of atheromatosis in cholesterol-fed rabbits. *J. Atherosclerosis Res. 7:* 343, 1967.

7. Kjeldsen, K.: *Smoking and atherosclerosis.* Copenhagen, Munksgaard, 1969.
8. Shepherd, J. T.: *Physiology of the circulation in human limbs in health and disease.* W. B. Saunders Company, Philadelphia and London, 1963.
9. Bollinger, A.: *Durchblutungsmessungen in der klinischen Angiologie.* Verlag Hans Huber, Bern und Stuttgart, 1969.
10. Hammond, E. C.: Smoking in relation to death rates of one million men and women. In *Epidemiological approaches to the study of cancer and other diseases* (ed. W. Haenzel). Bethesda, US Public Health Service, Natn. Cancer inst. Monogr. 19, 127–204, 1966.
11. Dahn, I.: On clinical use of venous occlusion plethysmography of calf. I. Methods and controls. *Acta chir. scand. 130*: 42, 1965.
12. Rose, G. A. and Blackburn, H.: Cardiovascular survey methods. WHO Monogr. Ser. 56: 1–188, 1968.
13. Dahn, I.: On clinical use of venous occlusion plethysmography of calf. II. Results in patients with arterial disease. *Acta chir. scand. 130*: 61, 1965.
14. Sternby, N. H.: Atherosclerosis in a defined population. An autopsy study in Malmö, Sweden. *Acta Path. et Microbiol. Scand.* Suppl. 194, 1968.

General discussion

Jerry Morris responded to the question Rose Stamler asked about how the IHD-register could be useful in studies of primary prevention. She believed that it is good for secondary but not for primary prevention. He said that the IHD-register could be used to assess end points for primary prevention!

Lars Wilhelmsen pointed out that all the risk factors from the prospective study of men born in 1913 in Gothenburg could be recognized in a clinical series of patients with myocardial infarction such as made available in an IHD-register.

Lars Werkö emphasized that a register will identify patients with all types of coronary heart diseases, including the cases of sudden death.

Geoffrey Rose noted that subjects with a family history of cardiovascular diseases have increased risk of a myocardial infarction. He underlined that this is of great practical importance because it is a piece of evidence that is available to the subjects themselves. At a practical level it is always very important to bear in mind that people whose fathers or other close relatives died of heart attacks are very often frightened and have in fact good reason to be so. Here is a group identified as being at high risk. Part of the explanation for this aggregation in families is genetic but it should be remembered also that habits tend to have familial aggregation.

Jerry Stamler wished to add one practical point. If one studies teenage children it is a mistake to dismiss the child if he shows a blood pressure reading that by usual clinical criteria falls within the normal range. The status of the parents should be considered also. What is very important is that the children of high risk parents tend to resemble their parents so that such children may need a stricter evaluation than other children.

From the audience someone asked what evidence we have that non-smoking normotensive subjects benefit from preventive measures?

Geoffrey Rose said that he thought there is no direct evidence and went on to say that most of the risk factors are not really simply present or absent from the prediction point of view. A »normotensive» person whose blood pressure is in the middle of the range of the blood pressure distribution of the population may well have a higher risk than a person with a lower than average pressure and this is similarly true for blood cholesterol. The common or population average blood pressure is by no means the ideal blood pressure and the same holds true for blood cholesterol. Theoretically, at least, we can believe that persons with only the »average» blood pressure and »average» cholesterol can reduce their risk of developing IHD by preventive measures.

Jerry Morris remarked that cerebrovascular diseases also are a world problem both in developed and in underdeveloped countries. The situation is quite different from that of ischaemic heart disease. Hypertension and cerebrovascular diseases are major problems in quite a number of developing countries.

Jerry Stamler said we should distinguish two questions of priority. One question concerns priorities within founds currently available for health services; the other has to do with priorities in the distribution of the whole G. N. P. He was very disturbed by any suggestion of abandoning, because of economic arguments, the classical Hippocratic humanitarian approach of medicine. The task of medicine is to apply to everyone the best of medical knowledge with no fancy talk of cost benefit analysis. The task of doctors is to demand application, on a world scale, of the best medical knowledge, the only consideration being that of the highest *medical* priority. Doctors must not allow themselves to be mesmerized by all kinds of considerations which end up by talking away money from health care. If doctors abandon the classical position of medicine they are in big trouble and will find themselves morally bankrupt.

Bertil Hood said that if we are to do high quality medical work the question is how many patients can we treat and what is the suitable age to intervene. He discussed genetically based screening in this connection. On the basis of patient records giving the worst possible family combination of hypertension, the younger siblings and the children of the propositus were invited for treatment. It was found that one could start at the age of thirty for practical purposes because it is still easy to bring the blood pressure down at that age. In hyperlipedemic disorders for the last twenty five years they had adopted a policy of attacking the risk factor as early as possible, at ages twenty to thirty.